ACADEMY FOR EDUCATIONAL DEVELOPMENT

Academy for Educational Development (AED) is an independent, nonprofit service organization committed to addressing human development needs in the United States and around the world through education, communication, and information. Under contracts and grants, the Academy operates programs for government and international agencies, educational institutions, foundations, and corporations. In partnership with its clients, AED focuses on increasing access to learning, improving the functioning of educational institutions, and expanding the sphere of education to support social and economic development.

AED offers a range of skills and services through three program divisions:

Social Development. Using innovative social marketing techniques, AED works with policy makers and practitioners in health, nutrition, family planning, and the environment to create communication and information systems to solve important social problems. AED is known as one of the leading institutions combining modern communication methodology and the social sciences to effect changes in health behavior, particularly through major international projects such as AIDSCOM, HealthCom, and Nutrition Communication programs in Africa, Asia, the Near East, Latin America, and the Caribbean.

Human Resources and Institutional Development. To support economic development, AED builds individual skills, strengthens training and academic institutions, and helps organizations capitalize on new skills.

Education and Exchange Services. Working with U.S. and international educators and policy makers, AED seeks to increase access to education and improve the performance of education systems to benefit people of all ages.

Last year, AED provided services in seventy-seven countries, including operation of thirty project field offices in twenty-three countries.

For additional information, please contact:

AED

Academy for Educational Development

ACADEMY FOR EDUCATIONAL DEVELOPMENT, INC.
Attn: Dr. William A. Smith, Executive Vice President
1255 Twenty-Third St., N.W.
Washington, D.C. 20037
(202) 862-1900

Communication for Health and Behavior Change

Judith A. Graeff
John P. Elder
Elizabeth Mills Booth

COMMUNICATION FOR HEALTH AND BEHAVIOR CHANGE

A Developing Country Perspective

Jossey-Bass Publishers
San Francisco

Manufactured in the United States of America on Lyons Falls Pathfinder Tradebook. This paper is acid-free and 100 percent totally chlorine-free.

The development of this document was an activity of HealthCom, or the Communication and Marketing for Child Survival Project. HealthCom is funded by the Office of Health in the Bureau for Research and Development, U.S. Agency for International Development (AID). HealthCom is conducted by the Academy for Educational Development (contract no. DPE-5984-Z-00-9018-00) and its subcontractors: the Center for International Health and Development Communication of the Annenberg School for Communication at the University of Pennsylvania, Applied Communication Technology, Birch & Davis International, The Futures Group, the Johns Hopkins University, and Porter/Novelli. This document does not necessarily represent the views or opinions of the U.S. Agency for International Development.

Credits are on page 205.

Library of Congress Cataloging-in-Publication Data

Graeff, Judith Allen.
Communication for health and behavior change : a developing country perspective / Judith A. Graeff, John P. Elder, Elizabeth Mills Booth. — 1st ed.
p. cm.—(The Jossey-Bass health series)
Prepared under the HealthCom project, Academy for Educational Development.
Includes bibliographical references and index.
ISBN 1-55542-585-2 (alk. paper)
1. Communication in medicine—Developing countries. 2. Health behavior—Research—Developing countries. 3. Health education—Developing countries. I. Elder, John P. II. Booth, Elizabeth Mills, date. III. HealthCom (Program) IV. Title. V. Series.
[DNLM: 1. Health Behavior. 2. Health Promotion. 3. Health Education. 4. Developing Countries. WA 395 G734c 1993]
R118.4.D44G73 1993
362.1'0425'091724—dc20
DNLM/DLC 93-26912
for Library of Congress CIP

FIRST EDITION
HB Printing 10 9 8 7 6 5 4 3 *Code 9391*

The Jossey-Bass Health Series

Contents

Tables, Figures, and Exhibits xiii

Preface xvii

The Authors xxv

1. Public Health in the Developing World 1

Child Health in Developing Countries • Child Survival Technologies • Health Communication for Child Survival • Health Communication, Culture, and Behavior Change • Applied Behavior Analysis: Myths and Reality • Summary

2. The ABCs of Behavior 19

Current Theories and Models of Health Behavior • Applied Behavior Analysis: Basic Terms • Summary

3. Assessing Behavior 37

Steps in Conducting Behavioral Assessment • Using Qualitative and Quantitative Research to Understand Consequences • Behavior Observation • Summary

4. Planning for Behavior Change 63

Selecting Target Behaviors • Selecting Communication Strategies • Selecting Communication Channels • Using Communication Channels as Consequences • Using Communication Channels in the A-B-C Chain • Summary

5. Skills Training 90

Using Behavioral Observation to Plan and Evaluate Training • Five Steps of Skills Training • Training as Reinforcement • Summary

6. Monitoring Behavior Change 109

Monitoring and Evaluation • Collecting Data for Monitoring • Graphing Monitoring Data • Reinforcing and Maintaining Behavior Change with Monitoring Data • Treating Monitoring as a Behavior • Summary

7. Maintaining Health Practices 131

Key Behavioral Principles • Program Implications • Assessing the Community and Health System for Sources of Support • Planning Communication Strategies for Maintenance • Other Maintenance-Related Communication Issues • Maintaining Initial Gains: The Honduran Example • Summary

8. Lessons and Implications for Future Work 150

Resource: The Communicator's Toolbox for Behavior Change 157

A. Performance Observation Checklist: Health Worker's Counseling Skills with Individual Mothers B. Performance Observation Checklist: Health Worker's Group Presentation Skills C. Ideal Behavior and Observation Checklist: Breast Feeding D. Performance Observation Checklist: Hand Washing E. Selecting Target Behaviors: The Behavior Analysis Scale F. Selecting Target Behaviors: Target Behavior Selection Worksheets G. Planning for Behavior Change Checklist H. Training for Behavior Change Checklist I. Monitoring for Behavior Change Checklist

References 185

Supplementary Reading 193

Index 195

Tables, Figures, and Exhibits

Tables

1.1. The History of the HealthCom Project 12

4.1. The Role of Communication Channels in the A-B-C Chain 86

4.2. Communication Strategies to Provide Antecedents and Consequences: Primary Audience—Mothers 87

4.3. Communication Strategies to Provide Antecedents and Consequences: Primary Audience—Health Workers 88

Figures

1.1. A Five-Step Methodology 15

2.1. Interactive Influences on Behavior as Viewed by Social Learning Theorists 25

2.2. Antecedents and Consequences of Behavior 33

4.1. Selecting Target Behaviors: Playing the Elimination Game 66

4.2. Selecting Communication Strategies: Decision Tree 73

5.1. Training and Feedback Loop 92

6.1. Number of Childhood Immunizations Given at Mumba Clinic, 1990–1992 119

6.2. Percentage of Clients Washing Hands Before Eating at Three Lunch Counters near La Plaza Market (Phase I) 121

6.3. Percentage of Clients Washing Hands Before Eating at Three Lunch Counters near La Plaza Market (Phase II) 123

6.4. Average Number of Diarrheal Disease Control Messages Fourteen Health Workers Used in Health Talks Pre/Post Training 124

6.5. Average Number of Communication Skills Fourteen Health Workers Used in Health Talks Pre/Post Training 125

6.6. Example of Self-Monitoring 127

7.1. Systems That Support Health Practices for Children 137

Exhibits

3.1. Ideal Behavior for ORT: Honduras Diarrheal Disease Control Program 40

3.2. Performance Observation: Mixing Oral Rehydration Solution 51

3.3. Narrative Observation: Immunizations in a Clinic 52

3.4. Clinic Frequency Observation 53

3.5. Clinic Duration Observation 55

3.6. Home ORS Administration Observation 56

3.7. A Growth-Monitoring Chart 57

5.1. Checklist for Evaluating Skills of Health Workers Counseling Mothers About Treatment for Children's Diarrhea 94

5.2. Checklist for Evaluating Health Workers' Skills After "Booster" Sessions 95

6.1. Vertical Axis of a Graph 116

6.2. Vertical and Horizontal Axes 117

6.3. A Completed Graph 118

Preface

Miriam lives in an urban shanty town with her husband and four children. She recently heard on the radio that today the neighborhood clinic is dispensing vaccines for childhood diseases. She prepares her nine-month-old infant for the journey and walks to the clinic through the crowded streets with her baby and her two-year-old child. The clinic is not open when she arrives, so Miriam waits with a few other women and children who have gathered there. When the health worker arrives, he takes care of the sick children first; so Miriam waits in the clinic until he has time for immunizations. These he does hastily, without checking for other problems that her children might have and without encouraging her to continue immunizing her baby through the completion of the series. Miriam leaves the clinic several hours after her arrival. Upon reaching home with her tired, cranky children, she finds her mother-in-law chatting with her husband while he is waiting for dinner. Her husband scolds her later for having neglected dinner and the other children for the sake of immunizing their healthy infant.

It is doubtful that Miriam will seek out further immunizations despite her conviction that they are important to her children's health. More information and motivation will not solve the problem for her or for the millions of women like her in developing countries. *Communication for Health and Behavior Change: A Developing Country Perspective* tells how health communication programs—besides providing information and motivation to caretakers—can teach skills and create an environment of support for behaviors critical to the health of children.

Millions of children in developing countries die every year from preventable diseases. In response, the international community has worked with governments, the health care delivery system, private organizations, and local communities to improve children's health. Because many of these deaths can be prevented, the role of health communication to teach and support preventive practices has become more and more central to public health programs in developing countries.

To get large-scale adoption of health practices to change morbidity and mortality rates has meant involving a broad range of people and systems. The implication for health communication is that behavior change takes more than just informing the public of the right thing to do. It takes applying a behavior change technology throughout the design and implementation of communication activities to produce some impact on a population's health practices.

Background

For nearly fifteen years, the Academy for Educational Development (AED), a private, nonprofit consulting firm, has implemented projects in health communication for child survival in developing countries. These projects have been funded by the United States Agency for International Development (USAID). AED has approached this task by working with local governments in applying a health communication methodology based on social marketing, anthropology, and applied behavior analysis. By following this methodology, program managers learn from the target audience the most culturally appropriate way to communicate desirable behavior change. They convert this information into effective health messages for interpersonal communication, broadcast media, and print materials; into skills-based training; and into programs to support health practices over time.

By focusing first on behavior change, AED found a good fit between the principles of applied behavior analysis and the communication methodology. The application of behavioral principles helped us analyze complex behaviors and the consequences to the people who performed them. This led to a communication strategy that considered the consequences and engaged positive events in individuals' environments to support them as they learned and adopted appropriate practices to improve children's health. The work described in this book, therefore, is a pioneering effort in health communication and in the application of behavior analysis to public health problems. We want to share this experience with others in the hope that readers will find some part of this experience in promoting child survival technologies in developing countries applicable to the health problems, the social and cultural context, and the target audiences they encounter.

Audience

Public health professionals from developing countries who seek further training in health communication in the West are surprised to find that few materials or courses are directly relevant to their primary concerns. In addition, professionals from industrialized nations who work in international health often find that the communication strategies that were successful in their own countries failed to achieve significant results when tried outside that context. This book is designed for those professionals—specifically, for all professionals working in health, family planning, and nutrition in developing countries who must design and manage communication components of public health programs. We use the term *communicator* in the text to refer to all these people involved in the communication process: physicians, program managers, health administrators, health educators, trainers, nurses, communications specialists, community workers, and others.

As mentioned, some of these health professionals are themselves from developing countries and are responsible for designing, managing, and evaluating health communication components of health programs. For example, in the public sector, professionals working in divisions of health education and health programs such as diarrheal disease control, family health, immunizations, maternal health, nutrition, and family planning have found this behavioral approach useful. Outside of the public sector, professionals in nongovernmental organizations, the media, and the commercial sector have also used this approach. Indeed, their experience has provided many of the illustrations described in the following chapters.

Communication for Health and Behavior Change is equally relevant for the range of professionals from industrialized nations who are involved in public health and communication overseas. The book shows them a theoretically based approach and tools that have been successfully applied in a variety of cultures and health areas.

Although written primarily to give practitioners a theoretical basis for their work in the field, the book can also serve as a text in a variety of training situations. Western schools of public health, for example, often draw 30 percent of their student body from developing countries; but these schools have few materials that are directly relevant to the priority health and communication issues those health professionals face in their work. This book would therefore be an excellent addition to materials discussed in public health schools' courses on international health, theories of health behavior, communication and health education, and social and cultural determinants of behavior. In addition, students of behavioral psychology, communication, and social marketing will find that the book opens a new field of application to their discipline. Finally, professional trainers should be able to apply many chapters of the book to their own work.

Overview of the Contents

Communication for Health and Behavior Change is more than a story of how-to-do-it-with-limited-resources. It explains behavioral analysis and its application to communication methodology in such a way that readers should be able to generalize the principles to their own work in other health areas or with different target audiences. The book shows, for example, how this approach was used to change behaviors other than health behaviors. The approach was used to change and maintain the practice of health communication itself—by teaching and supporting effective interpersonal communication skills in health workers. Thus, the book shows that the same principles used to train and support mothers' skills have broad application to general behavioral issues throughout the health system.

Chapter One gives an overview of high-priority child health issues in developing countries and briefly describes the essential health technologies and communication methodology currently being used to respond to those issues. The chapter includes a description of how internationally coordinated work is conducted in child survival and how one organization's experience formed the basis for the book.

Chapter Two briefly describes several relevant psychological theories before describing applied behavior analysis. This chapter is intended to ground readers in certain principles of applied behavior analysis. It defines the behavioral terms and concepts critical to understanding why certain approaches are taken, strategies developed, or tools used in the communication programs described in later chapters.

Chapters Three to Seven follow the steps of health communication methodology—assess, plan, train, monitor, and maintain—and present the applicable behavioral concepts and tools at each step. Each chapter gives examples of how these concepts and tools were used in actual child survival communication activities.

Chapter Three, on behavioral assessment, shows readers how to use behavioral principles to describe the ideal behavior and to determine what behaviors the target audience is already performing, what competing behaviors it might be performing, and what events (antecedents and consequences) influence the occurrence of those behaviors. Readers also learn how to apply behavioral observation as an aid in the assessment process.

Chapter Four, on planning for behavior change, takes the information gained in assessment and shows how to use it to select target behaviors. Readers are led through the elimination process to identify a few target behaviors for communication that are feasible for the target audience to do, have the most potential impact on health, and are the most amenable to change and adoption.

The chapter on skills training (Chapter Five) presents five steps necessary for the trainees' mastery of target behaviors: instructions, demonstration, practice, feedback, and homework with feedback. The use of direct behavioral observation is stressed, as well as the importance of constructive and rewarding feedback in helping the trainee acquire and maintain the skill. Training sessions themselves, as the chapter demonstrates, can function as positive consequences to participants in health communication programs and become a key component to sustaining behavior change over the long term.

The chapter on monitoring (Chapter Six) emphasizes two main points. First, progress toward the learning and adoption of target behaviors can and should be measured throughout the life of a program. Techniques described are direct observation, the use of clinical and other records, and self-monitoring. Second, monitoring data, used as feedback on personal or program performance, can function as a positive consequence to participants. Thus, monitoring results themselves, if presented as feedback in a constructive and simple (visual) form, can help strengthen the very behaviors being measured.

Chapter Seven discusses how programs can use behavioral principles to maintain individual health practices over the long term. To date, communication programs in developing countries have been limited in applying these principles, so the tone of this chapter is forward looking—describing what programs will need to do to sustain the behavior changes achieved so far. The basic idea is that without support from the broad social environment, health practices—especially preventive ones—are unlikely to be maintained over the long term. In this chapter, we continue to focus on observable behavior of individuals and actions of organizations and describe ways of "finding an environment of support for target behavior." Communicators first identify individuals and organizations in the target audience's community, social, and political environment that can provide reinforcement and feedback for target behaviors. Behavioral principles can then be applied in successfully engaging selected individuals and organizations to support health practices over time.

The book closes with a chapter on what we and others learned from applying behavior analysis in health communication for child survival. This chapter, Chapter Eight, suggests further directions for those working for health behavior change in developing countries. It also discusses implications for work in industrialized nations as the world grows more and more into a global community.

The "Communicator's Toolbox" resource at the end of the book provides readers with many of the instruments described in the text. These checklists, forms, and scales are to be viewed as demonstrations of behaviorally based instruments. Readers interested in using them should carefully adapt the instruments to fit a specific health or cultural context.

Acknowledgments

Many people helped set the stage for the perspective and experiences described in this book. Anthony Meyer, USAID, developed the Mass Media for Health Practices and HealthCom I project, creating the mandate to explore the interrelationship of communication, behavior change, and public health in developing countries. Robert Clay continued that mandate in later HealthCom work. William Smith and the behavioral consultants Paul Touchette, Douglas Porter, John Elder, Scott Geller, and James Holland provided the intellectual and behavioral leadership on the projects, especially in their formative years.

We would like to acknowledge the contributions of Scott Geller to the chapter on training, of Dennis Foote and Carol Baume to the chapter on maintenance, and of Sylvia Lopez Gaona to the introduction. Thanks go to the staff of Technologies for Primary Health Care, Larry Casazza, Eileen Hanlon and Karen White, for their technical assistance with the child survival technologies, and to Anita Menon for her help with referencing. A special thank-you goes to the panel of reviewers whose thoughtful comments helped to shape the document: Soulimane Baro, Karin Bergstrom, Tarcisio Carneiro, Eleanora de Guzman, Scott Geller, Deborah Helitzer-

Allen, Wilma Meeus, Douglas Porter, Mark Rasmuson, Thomas Reis, Renata Seidel, William Smith, and Paul Touchette. We also thank Maria Claudia De Valdenebro for her fine work on the graphics used throughout the book. Diane Mason's patience and thoroughness throughout the long process of manuscript preparation in Washington, D.C., are greatly appreciated. Amelia Arroyo and Anna Morghen did fine work in coordinating the preparation of drafts and communication with Washington and Kansas from San Diego.

We also humbly recognize the dedication, energy, and wisdom of the hundreds of health and communication professionals in Latin America, Africa, and Asia who worked closely with project staff and consultants to help bring about changes necessary to save children's lives.

Reader Feedback

We are interested in your reactions and suggestions. We invite you to share your general ideas regarding style, format, and content, as well as any specific suggestions regarding confusions, additions, elisions, and so on. It would help if we knew a bit about you and how you used the book to design a communication program, a training workshop, or a component of your curriculum. In addition, if you develop instructional materials, we would love to see them. Send your feedback to Judith A. Graeff, Academy for Educational Development, 1255 23d St., NW, Washington, D.C., 20037.

August 1993

Judith A. Graeff
Washington, D.C.

John P. Elder
La Mesa, California

Elizabeth Mills Booth
Lawrence, Kansas

The Authors

Judith A. Graeff is currently senior program officer for the HealthCom project at the Academy for Educational Development. She received her B.A. degree (1970) from the University of Michigan in psychology; her Ph.D. degree (1979) from the State University of New York at Stony Brook in behavioral clinical psychology; and her M.P.H. degree (1986) from the Johns Hopkins University School of Hygiene and Public Health in international health. Since 1987, Graeff has managed the behavioral research component of the HealthCom project, as well as managing health communication activities in several of HealthCom's African sites. Starting as a Peace Corps volunteer in Côte d'Ivoire, she has lived and worked overseas for seven years.

John P. Elder is currently a professor in the Graduate School of Public Health at San Diego State University, where he is head of the Division of Health Promotion. He received his B.A. degree (1974) from the University of Nebraska in psychology; his Ph.D. degree (1978) from West Virginia University in behavioral psychology; and his M.P.H. degree (1984) from Boston University in health administration. Elder has published extensively in areas such as behavior modification, epidemiology and chronic disease prevention, and child survival. Working with the Academy for Educational Development and other firms, he has helped implement and evaluate health projects and conduct behavioral research in ten different Latin American, Asian, and other developing countries. He currently is funded by the National Institutes of Health for a project that integrates health promotion materials into English as a Second Language classes for recent immigrants.

Elizabeth Mills Booth is a health communication and social marketing specialist who has worked in more than twenty countries in the developing world. For fifteen of the last twenty years, she has lived in Latin America and Africa. She received her B.A. degree (1972) from Kansas State University in journalism and mass communication, and her M.A. degree (1977) from Indiana University in education. Booth has worked for the Academy for Educational Development since 1979, beginning as assistant field director of the Mass Media and Health Practices project in Honduras and continuing in management positions with the HealthCom project. She was one of the first to use communication to change and support behaviors related to oral rehydration therapy. She is presently consultant to the Academy for Educational Development and other clients, including the World Health Organization, the Pan American Health Organization, the Nutrition Institute for Central America and Panama, the Johns Hopkins University, the Kellogg Foundation, and KWSO Radio, Oregon.

Communication for Health and Behavior Change

1

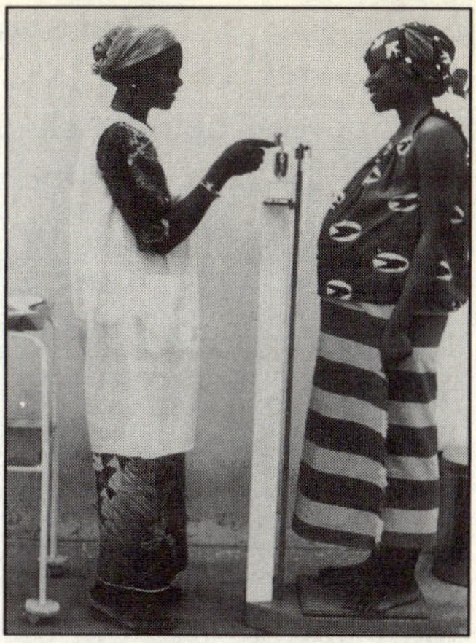

Public Health in the Developing World

In the time it takes you to read this sentence, one hundred children throughout the world will have died. More than two thousand children die every minute in the developing world, almost three million children every day. Most of these deaths could be prevented by better living conditions, widespread literacy, less crowding, and less civil strife. Much suffering and death could also be prevented with the appropriate use of simple health technologies such as oral rehydration salts, timely immunizations, and growth monitoring; and the introduction and support of breast feeding, diarrhea prevention, infant weaning, and other health practices. Increasingly, health professionals in both developing and industrialized countries are realizing that in order to reduce morbidity and mortality, we need to go beyond developing health systems' infrastructure and "educating" the public. We need to change and support what people actually *do* about their own and their children's health.

The authors have been fortunate to be part of a pioneering effort in public health, communication, and behavior change in the developing world. We have worked with talented and committed health professionals from industrialized and developing countries in an effort to learn how a behavioral approach to health communication can help us change and support health practices. As we worked together over the years, we found that providing information was not enough. We needed to focus more directly on actual behavior change. At first, we emphasized mothers' and other caretakers' behavior, but we found that we needed to apply the same approach concurrently to the behavior of other people: the village health worker, clinic staffs, and of the people working throughout the entire Ministry of Health system. This book is a reflection of our experience.

As we talked with people about our work, both in the United States and throughout the world, we found that they often wanted more background in order to put our experience in an understandable context. Some people are not familiar with the health problems in developing countries and the international community's role in supporting solutions to those problems. Others wonder how organizations such as the Academy for Educational Development work in a country: whom do we work with, and how are communities approached and involved? Some people are not familiar with the recent experience and advancements in health communication. Many are unfamiliar with or have misconceptions about the theory of behavior analysis and its contribution to health communication. This introduction attempts to answer these questions and give readers a common ground for understanding the story that *Communication for Health and Behavior Change* tells.

Child Health in Developing Countries

Just over one-third of the people in most developing countries are under the age of fifteen; so maternal-child health, child survival, and family planning usually predominate in the public health agenda of those countries (United Nations, 1991). As a result, the control and prevention of infectious diseases affecting children dominate health programming. The treatment and prevention of diarrheal disease, malaria, measles, and acute respiratory infections are among the major interventions. Since the interrelationship between disease and malnutrition is a critical risk factor in developing countries, breast feeding, appropriate weaning practices, and dietary increases in important micronutrients such as vitamin A, iodine, and iron are also saving lives. Family-planning programs are important because high-risk fertility behaviors have a direct impact on the survival of children. Because the spread of AIDS is a critical factor in child survival as well as that of adults, AIDS programs have major implications for the health and well-being of children.

Certain other demographic factors have important implications for designing and implementing public health programs in developing countries. As more of the population emigrates to urban centers, rapid urbanization is breaking down traditional social structures to the point where usual support systems are no longer functioning effectively. Overcrowding and poverty increase the risk for the spread of infectious disease. In many countries, economic underdevelopment has led to a relatively weak health infrastructure that cannot meet the needs of rapid population growth. Health facilities are often scarce, supplies erratic, and hospital staff underpaid and overworked. Public health programs can help people prevent disease and use simple treatments at home to relieve the burden on the health infrastructure. Despite significant increases in literacy in the last ten years, an average of only 68 percent of men and 50 percent of women in developing countries can read (Holmes & Aral, 1991). Functional literacy rates in many countries are actually much lower, especially in rural areas. Low literacy rates have important implications for health communication programs because large portions of the population are not accustomed to learning from print and visual materials, even if the materials do not contain words. Because most developing countries have a variety of cultural, ethnic, and linguistic groups within their borders, the same health message often cannot be understood nationwide.

Health professionals in developing countries, faced with this demographic context and these priority health problems, are asking questions such as these:

> "How can my diarrheal disease control program increase better feeding practices as well as decrease deaths caused by dehydration?"
>
> "My data show that bottle feeding is still practiced in urban areas. What changes can we make in hospital policy and

practices to encourage and train mothers to breast-feed when they leave the maternity ward?"

"What institutional changes are necessary to sustain the 70 percent immunization coverage achieved in my country?"

"Clinic health workers don't seem to be very effective in their health education efforts. How can I help them communicate better with mothers?"

"More and more women with children are contracting AIDS every year. What can I do to encourage couples to use condoms, and what support can I give to families who have ill mothers?"

"A large proportion of young children are malnourished in this country despite the general availability of food and little civil strife. How can I get parents to seek out and feed more nourishing food to their children?"

"Nearly all the women in this region are giving birth at home without an attendant or any prenatal care. What can our staff do to increase women's usage of our clinic's prenatal and delivery services?"

There is no one solution for any of these problems. Much can be done, however, if individuals, communities, and people in the health system work together to change health and professional practices. This broad environment of support for children's health and well-being could have an actual impact on morbidity and mortality. Considering the financial, human and infrastructure resources available, the challenge to create and sustain such an environment seems daunting.

Child Survival Technologies

In 1978, the World Health Organization (WHO) and the United Nations Children's Fund (UNICEF) sponsored the International Conference on Primary Health Care in Alma-Ata, Kazakhstan. Experts from developing and industrialized countries worked together to draft a ten-part declaration that became the blueprint for international primary health care and public health during the 1980s. An outgrowth of this declaration was the identification of a package of child survival technologies and behaviors with the potential for reducing infant mortality in priority health areas. Participants at the 1990 World Summit for Children, held at the United Nations, promised to continue to reduce child deaths and child malnutrition. They drew up a Convention on the Rights of the Child, which was ratified by over one hundred nations. Included in its purpose are specific goals for improving child health. The HealthCom project worked in a number of those targeted health areas: diarrheal disease control, immunizable diseases, acute respiratory infections, infant and child nutrition, malaria, and high-risk fertility.

Diarrheal Disease Control

Diarrheal disease is one of the leading causes of infant and child mortality in the world today. An estimated three million children die from diarrhea every year (United Nations Children's Fund, 1992). The primary means of preventing death from dehydration and other complications from diarrheal disease is oral rehydration therapy (ORT). This form of treatment was taught to one-third of the developing world's families in the 1980s and is now preventing over one million child deaths each year (World Health Organization, Programme for Control of Diarrheal Diseases, 1990). It involves increasing fluids and continuing feeding at the onset of diarrhea. If diarrhea persists or the stools become bloody or contain mucus, help should be sought from a professional health care facility. Fluids can be obtained in the form of a prepackaged mixture of oral rehydration salts (ORS), which are available at little or no cost from pharmacies, health facilities, and networks of community distributors. A properly prepared, home-based sugar-salt solution and other recommended fluids available in the home also can be used. Continuation of feeding—including breast feeding and rice- or cereal-based gruels—during diarrheal episodes can protect a child's nutritional status and may shorten the period of illness. Practices in the prevention of diarrhea include exclusive breast feeding for the first four to six months of life; immunization against measles; and basic hygiene practices such as hand washing, sanitary disposal of feces, and the use of clean drinking water.

The recent pandemic of cholera, one of various types of diarrheal disease, has caused great concern in Latin America, Asia, and Africa. Cholera is particularly dangerous because it rapidly progresses to the state of severe dehydration. Since wage-earning adults can be affected as well as children, this form of diarrhea causes significant economic and political problems. The preventive measures, however, are much like those for other diarrheal diseases. Between 80 and 90 percent of cholera cases can be rehydrated through oral rehydration (World Health Organization, Programme for Control of Diarrheal Diseases, 1991). The key is to administer the treatment as early in the episode as possible.

Immunizable Diseases

An estimated 1.7 million infants and children die from infectious diseases: measles, diphtheria, pertussis, tetanus, and tuberculosis. Another 120,000 cases of paralytic poliomyelitis occur every year (World Health Organization, 1991). The primary effort toward universal protection from these diseases is the worldwide Expanded Programme of Immunization (EPI). With the current 80 percent immunization coverage rate reported in the last decade, an estimated 3.2 million child deaths are being prevented per year. Full immunization for children includes a series of vaccinations. The mother is vaccinated during pregnancy for neonatal tetanus. The child is vaccinated at birth with BCG (Bacillus of Calmette and Guérin for tuberculosis); at six, ten, and fourteen weeks for DPT (diphtheria, pertussis, and tetanus) and polio; and at nine months for measles.

A number of obstacles can prevent health workers from administering and caretakers and parents from completing the series of immunizations. Vaccines produced can be of low quality. Storage facilities and transportation can be inadequate; as a result, the "cold chain" for vaccines can be broken (that is, they are not maintained at adequately refrigerated levels), thus lowering the vaccines' effectiveness. If a child is feverish, health workers or caretakers often decide against vaccination. The side effects produced by some vaccinations may discourage caretakers from returning for the remainder of the series. Health care facilities can be hard to reach or overcrowded, causing caretakers to be away from the household for long periods of time; thus, other children may be left unattended and the household duties unfinished. Despite these obstacles, through careful production, distribution, and communication with health care providers and caretakers, many countries are increasing immunization coverage yearly.

Acute Respiratory Infections

From 25 to 30 percent of all deaths in infants and young children in the developing world are attributable to acute respiratory infections (ARI). An estimated four million children succumb to these infections every year (World Health Organization, Programme for Control of Acute Respiratory Infections, 1990). Unfortunately, no single, low-cost technology exists for preventing ARI or treating children who have these infections. At present, treatment calls for increasing liquids, clearing the nose, and continuing feeding during mild episodes (the common cold). When cases become severe, mothers should seek assistance from a health care facility. It is at this stage that many cases of severe ARI (usually pneumonia) become deadly because of inappropriate household response. Often caretakers will continue the use of home remedies, delay in seeking medical help, comply poorly with recommended therapy, or fail to recognize the signs of pneumonia. For this reason, it is vital for caretakers to recognize when an infection has progressed from being manageable in the home to requiring trained health care. Health workers should be adequately trained in detecting severe cases of ARI, in case management, and in the appropriate use of medication.

Infant and Child Nutrition

Malnutrition is too often the common denominator of the disease and deprivation processes that threaten child survival. Undernutrition affects nearly 40 percent of all children in developing countries. It contributes directly and indirectly to an estimated 60 percent of all child deaths (United States Agency for International Development, 1991). When a child is malnourished, his or her immune system is weakened and unable to ward off infection. Disease, in turn, can contribute to malnutrition. Children who survive this cycle lack the nutritional stores to reach their full mental and physical growth potential. Apart from inadequate food production and distribution systems and low family-income levels, a major factor in poor nutrition is inappropriate family feeding practices. Caretakers must continue feeding children nutritious foods during episodes of disease despite the lack of appetite.

Proper feeding is also crucially linked to breast feeding and weaning. A child should be exclusively breast-fed for the first four to six months of life. During the weaning period, the new diet should be introduced gradually and should contain foods that are high in nutritional value, provide sufficient calories, and can be easily digested. Traditional weaning foods, however, are excessively bulky for infants to consume in sufficient quantities, and these foods often do not contain adequate calories and nutrients. The results of unsuccessful weaning can be seen on growth charts used in growth-monitoring programs. Caretakers periodically have their children's weight measured and recorded at a health facility. Drops in growth or inadequate growth can be tracked, enabling health workers to identify nutritional problems before they reach dangerous stages. Health workers, in turn, must be able to communicate with caretakers about these nutritional problems and the feasible feeding practices that can bring about improvement.

In addition to regular feeding practices, micronutrient supplements play an important role in child nutritional health. The most common are iron, iodine, and vitamin A. Iron deficiency is the leading cause of anemia, which affects 40 percent of the developing world's children and 50 percent of pregnant women (United States Agency for International Development, 1991). The lack of iron undermines the health of the body's immune system and therefore increases the risk of infection. Infants born to anemic mothers have low birthweights and are at a greater risk of mortality. Iron-rich foods and iron supplements are recommended to prevent anemia in adults and children. Iodine deficiency in pregnant mothers can cause mental retardation in infants. Presently, the most common intervention is for governments to iodize salt supplies. Vitamin A deficiency is the leading cause of childhood blindness. An estimated five to ten million children in the developing world show signs (visual impairment) of deficiency in vitamin A. The lack of vitamin

A can also contribute to the overall health of the child. Children who are deficient are more prone to infections, experience longer episodes of infection and are more likely to die from these infections than are children who receive supplements (United States Agency for International Development, 1991). Families are being encouraged to include more vitamin A-rich foods in their diet when available, and to grow green, leafy vegetables. Vitamin A programs are attempting to introduce vitamin A-rich foods in areas where these foods are not available and to administer vitamin A capsules or liquids once very six months to children between one and five years of age and to mothers in the first month after delivery.

Malaria

Malaria is one of the farthest-reaching diseases in the world today. Over half the world's population lives in areas where it is found, and an estimated 250 to 300 million cases occur every year. Most of the cases (80 percent) occur in sub-Saharan Africa, where one million children die from malaria every year (United States Agency for International Development, 1991). The disease is transmitted by the female anopheles mosquito and by mothers to children through the placenta. The parasite attacks red blood cells, causing anemia and complications with the spleen, kidney, and brain. Symptoms include fever, chills, diarrhea, nausea, profuse sweating, muscle pain, and prostration. All these symptoms can be especially dangerous to a young child because they can lead to dehydration, malnutrition, and an increased susceptibility to infection. For the prevention and treatment of malaria, drugs such as chloroquine and mefloquine are administered. Treatment is complicated, however, when strains of malaria become resistant to chloroquine, as they have in some fifty five countries (United States Agency for International Development, 1991), or when caretakers prematurely cease to administer the drugs because adverse side effects appear or because the drugs cause the symptoms to disappear before the disease is actually overcome. Besides drug treatment, other recommended treatment measures include improving diagnostic equipment in health facilities and enhancing the ability of health workers to detect the symptoms of malaria. Communities can help to prevent malaria by draining ditches and planting trees in swamps, thereby destroying the breeding grounds. The primary means of prevention, however, is the use of insecticides in massive spraying. Spraying nets hung over beds with insecticide has also proven effective. Families can be directly involved in prevention by wearing protective clothing and using screens where available.

High-Risk Fertility

The risks involved in fertility lie in three categories: age of mother, number of children borne, and length of time between births. Infant mortality rates based on mother's age are highest with teenaged mothers and then with older mothers. The younger or older a mother is, the higher the risk for the mother and the child. When a woman gives birth to more than four children, the health risk to mother and child becomes greater with every subsequent child. The greatest risk factor, however, is in births that are spaced less than two years apart. The infant mortality rate for children born at intervals of less than two years is 71 percent higher than for children born at two- to three-year intervals (United States Agency for International Development, 1991). Children born under high-risk circumstances experience inhibited growth patterns and heightened risk of infection, usually because they are unable to overcome low birthweight.

The health of the mother is also threatened with every type of high-risk birth; and her poor health, in turn, inhibits her ability to care for the rest of her children. Information, education, and communication programs are one of the primary means of lowering the incidence of high-risk births. Family-planning services encourage exclusive breast feeding, promote birth spacing, and provide women with the technology and information needed for contraception.

Health Communication for Child Survival

As can be seen, child survival requires that individuals at many levels of the social structure—the home, the community, and the health system—work together to change their practices related to children's health. To have an impact, these practices need to be carried out correctly and in a timely fashion. During the 1970s and 1980s, several theories of behavior change emerged and were subsequently used in industrialized countries to combat chronic disease. Theory-based interventions were applied in public health programs to change high-risk life-styles, such as smoking, high-fat diets, and lack of exercise. The question remained, however, whether such theory-based approaches were applicable to the priority health issues and demographic and cultural context of developing countries. If so, how would these approaches translate into public health programs?

In the 1980s, international donor agencies and the governments of developing countries began exploring the role of health communication to introduce and support child survival technologies and practices. The United States Agency for International Development (USAID) funded a series of five-year projects to work with professionals in developing countries, in an effort to create and refine a health communication methodology adapted to their priority health issues and demographic and cultural contexts. The Academy for Educational Development (AED), an independent, nonprofit organization, has carried out these projects. The project was initially called Mass Media for Health Practices (MMHP). Its mandate was not only to promote healthy behavior but also to develop a communication methodology, understand why it worked, and transfer it to local institutions.

MMHP initially promoted ORT in Honduras and The Gambia, and then expanded to other countries and child survival technologies. In five years, MMHP became "Communication for Child Survival" (HealthCom). The changing title reflects a growing sophistication in the approach to the role that human behavior plays in maintaining human health. Indeed, HealthCom's mandate was to test the role of behavior analysis in the communication methodology. Over the past twelve years, HealthCom has worked in more than twenty countries to promote a variety of child survival technologies. A description of the project can be found in a 1992 publication, *Results and Realities: A Decade of Experience in Communication for Child Survival,* available from AED. Table 1.1 summarizes the scope of MMHP and HealthCom's experience.

Generally, the HealthCom project works by sending a "res-

Table 1.1. The History of the HealthCom Project.

	Child Survival Technology							
Country and Period of Project	*CDD*	*EPI*	*M*	*ARI*	*Vit. A*	*BF*	*GM*	*FP*
Burkina Faso, 1992–1993		X						
Ecuador, 1983–1990	X	X					X	X
The Gambia, 1981–1984	X							
Guatemala, 1986–1990	X	X						
Honduras, 1980–1992	X	X	X	X			X	X
Indonesia, 1985–1993	X	X			X			
Jordan, 1987–1989						X		
Lesotho, 1986–1990	X	X				X		X
Malawi, 1986–1988	X	X	X					
Mali, 1991–1992	X	X						X
Mexico, 1986–1992	X							
Nigeria, 1987–1990	X	X	X					
Papua New Guinea, 1988–1990	X							
Paraguay, 1987–1990	X					X		
Peru, 1983–1990	X	X						X
Philippines, 1987–1990	X	X		X				
Senegal, 1991–1993	X	X	X					X
Swaziland, 1984–1985	X							
Yemen, 1988–1992	X	X						
Zaire, 1988–1990	X	X	X					

CDD—control of diarrheal disease, EPI—immunization, M—malaria, ARI—acute respiratory infection, BF—breast feeding, GM—growth monitoring, FP—family planning.

ident adviser" to live in a specific country for the life of the project—usually two to four years. Resident advisers frequently call on short-term technical assistance to assist them in providing training and technical support to the communication activities in the country. The resident adviser works primarily with the Ministry of Health's Division of Health Education and the head of appropriate health programs, such as family health, immunization, or diarrheal disease control. At the same time, HealthCom staff support ministry goals of decentralization by providing training and communication support to regional Ministry of Health personnel, hospital and clinic staff, and primary health care workers. Depending on the country context and infrastructure, the HealthCom staff assist the ministry in identifying and working with other local groups and institutions, such as private voluntary organizations, advertising agencies, research firms, schools of public health, nursing schools, and radio and television stations. Community groups are also often engaged to introduce and support practices and products. For example, the Indonesian Ministry of Health works with national women's organizations, whose approximately 450,000 members include women from virtually every town and village. In each setting, the role of the HealthCom staff is to train their counterparts in developing countries to conduct their communication work more systematically and effectively. (For a description of an immunization communication program, see Verzosa, Bernaje, de Guzman, Hernandez, Reodica, & Taguiwalo, 1989.)

Health Communication, Culture, and Behavior Change

Health communication is the systematic attempt to influence positively the health practices of large populations. The primary goal of health communication is to bring about improvements in health-related practices and, in turn, health status. Although many professionals working in this area make a distinction among the terms *health education; health communication; health promotion;* and *information, education, and communication* (IEC), there is a great deal of overlap in actual practice, and in this book we will not make distinctions among these terms. We use the word *communicator* to refer not only to those specifically trained in these areas but also to any public health professional involved in changing health behavior through communication programs.

Effective health communication is a combination of art and science. Nevertheless, one of the keys to success is the application of a scientific and systematic health communication methodology to public health problems. Although the actual communication strategies HealthCom helped to develop were strikingly different from country to country, the methodology employed was similar and was critical in making communication programs truly reflect the needs and cultural context of each country.

Health communicators agree that the communication process must alternate listening and doing—research and action. The communicator enters into a dialogue with the community through the use of ongoing systematic research with representatives of the target audience. We first listen to the community during assessment, in order to plan communication strategies and activities based on that community's needs, cultural context, and practices. We then test sample strategies and materials with the community before delivering them on a mass scale. After a period of time, we use focused research to listen to the community and, on the basis of community members' reactions, change and fine-tune the communication strategies and activities if necessary. This combination of research and action "puts the client in the driver's seat," making the communication strategies respond specifically to the client's needs. In this book, the communication methodology includes five steps: assess, plan, pretest, deliver, and monitor (Rasmuson, Seidel, Smith, & Booth, 1988). (See Figure 1.1.)

This approach to health communication is derived from various disciplines, including social marketing, anthropology, behavior analysis, advertising, communication, education, and other social sciences. These disciplines complement each other and share common principles and techniques; yet each one makes a unique contribution to the health communication methodology. Of these, anthropology, social marketing, and behavioral analysis predominate the methodology. Anthropology helps the planner (whether in a Ministry of Health, a private corporation, or a community group) understand the cultural characteristics, including the beliefs and practices, of a population, in order to offer programs consistent with the values and language of the target audience. Social marketing provides a process for developing creative strategies to promote health practices and products. This book will focus on the contribution that applied behavior analysis has made in health communication.

Applied Behavior Analysis: Myths and Reality

"Behavior analysis is a behavioral science that develops and experimentally analyzes practical procedures for producing change in socially significant behaviors" (Baer, Wolf, & Risley, 1968, p. 91)—or, less formally, behavior analysis is a discipline that studies the relationships between behavior and the (interpersonal or physical) environment and modifies these relationships in such a way as to help an individual adopt new and more functional behaviors

Figure 1.1. A Five-Step Methodology.

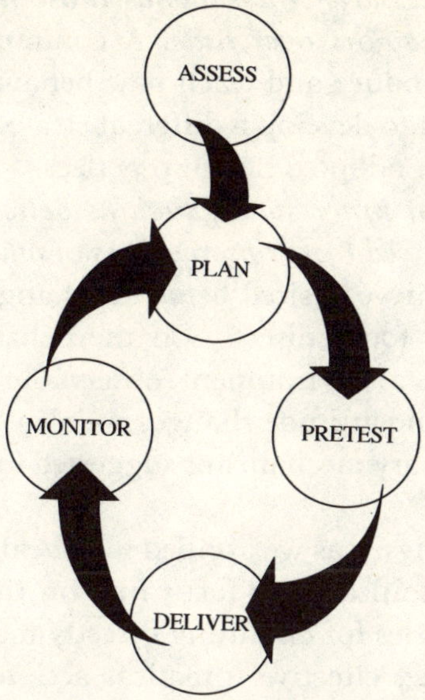

Source: HealthCom brochure, 1991. Published by the Academy for Educational Development, Washington, DC. Reprinted with permission.

(Elder, Geller, Hovell, & Mayer, 1993). Four principles of behavior analysis are particularly relevant to health communication:

1. *Most behavior is learned within a cultural, socioeconomic, and individual context and therefore can be relearned or unlearned, or new behaviors can be introduced.* Individuals can learn to adopt new health practices and make their current ones more effective.
2. *Behavior, including health-related behavior, is shaped by events and reactions (antecedents and consequences) in the social and physical environment.* When these conditions change, the person's behavior is also likely to change. A communication strategy that helps a population move toward better health does so by using antecedents and consequences to change and maintain appropriate practices. Organizations as well as individuals can help to create this environment of support for health practices.

3. *Environmental conditions necessary for learning new behaviors are not necessarily the same as those necessary for maintaining the behaviors over time.* A communication program designed to introduce and teach new behaviors to a target audience will need to develop a different strategy to provide long-term support for adopted health practices.
4. *The existence of inner states, such as beliefs and knowledge, can only be inferred from observations of what people do or say they do.* To achieve desired behavior change, communication programs must focus directly on the behavior itself and the social and physical environment (observable events) supporting it. Knowledge and attitude changes are also of interest, but they are not the primary mechanisms suggested for behavior change.

Behavior analysis, as we applied it in health communication for child survival, helped us to focus first on the desired behavior and to design strategies for obtaining directly measurable results. It suggested immediate, effective, practical action to use in all the steps of the health communication methodology. Approaching health communication from a behavioral perspective gave us a basis for examining the close relationship between a health behavior and the events preceding and following it. We put a microscope on complex health practices and described how they are influenced by the social and cultural environment. Specifically, we were better able to understand the environments in which behaviors operated and to identify culturally appropriate health and community systems to support healthy behavior.

There are many misconceptions and stereotypes concerning behavior analysis. Some people believe that it is a mechanistic, antidemocratic approach; that it manipulates the individuals supposedly being served by a program; and that behavior analysts hold secrets to behavior control unknown to the general (and innocent) public. However, as the discipline has developed, a wide variety of professionals and nonprofessionals have adapted and used its principles and techniques. During the twelve years of the HealthCom project, health professionals in over twenty countries, from program directors to clinic workers, have learned to use these principles to help their communities adopt healthier life-styles.

Others believe that behavior analysis is simplistic or "reductionistic." Because it relies primarily on observing and measuring individual behavior, it seems to ignore mental processes and social and cultural influences. Although behavior analysis does focus on the behavior of individuals, the solutions it suggests incorporate the wider environment and therefore include cultural influences, social norms, and community involvement in changing and maintaining behavior. Principles and techniques from social marketing and anthropology assist the communicator in incorporating social and cultural influences on behavior into planning and implementation of communication programs.

In our experience, people who are unaware of or ignore these stereotypes, or who are not tied to any one theory of communication and behavior, have found behavior analysis useful in their daily work. Professionals from anthropology or social marketing, for example, have used many skills-training or reinforcement-based interventions in communication programs. Professionals in the fields of health education, community medicine, or agricultural extension appreciate the direct, behavioral measurement approach of behavior analysis. In the HealthCom experience, this interdisciplinary melting pot has influenced and refined the professional approaches of both behavior analysts and their counterparts from other disciplines.

Summary

Health communication has had a significant role in changing behaviors related to child survival, especially in the areas of diarrheal disease control and immunization in a variety of cultural settings throughout the developing world (see, for example, Baume, 1990; Elder, Boddy, Barriga, Aguilar, & Espinal, 1991; Elder, et al., 1992; Hornik, Contreras-Budge, Ferencic, Koepke, & Morris, 1991; Hornik, Zimicki, & Lee, 1991; McDivitt & McDowell, 1991; Touchette, Elder, & Naigel, 1990). These experiences have demonstrated that communication, in coordination with communities and the health care delivery system, can produce significant behavior change in a target population.

Behavior analysis has provided a useful approach, tools, and techniques to introduce new behaviors and technologies. The question now being asked is what role this behavioral approach to communication can play in maintaining these positive changes. Successful experience in initiating behavior change suggests that behavior analysis will also be useful in helping communicators develop strategies to maintain positive health practices. Future health communication programs will test how effective behaviorally based strategies are in maintaining health practices over time.

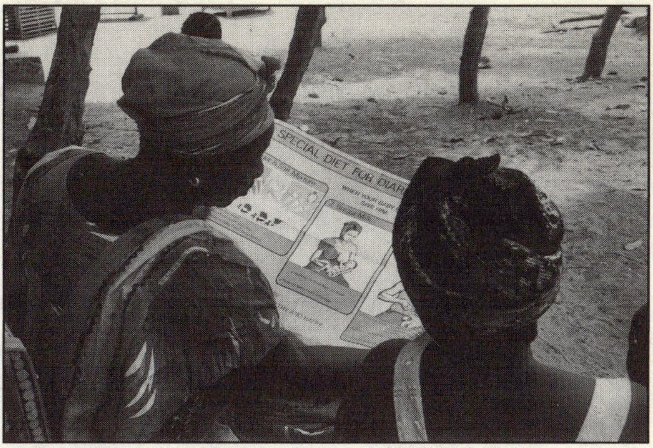

2

The ABCs of Behavior

Health communication has been defined as "the modification of human behavior and environmental factors related to that behavior which directly or indirectly promote health, prevent illness or protect individuals from harm" (Elder, Geller, Hovell, & Mayer, in press). With roots in education and health education, the field of health communication is now heavily influenced by psychology, communication, and other behavioral science disciplines. Corresponding to this preeminence is the dominance of psychologically based theories and models of health behavior.

Current Theories and Models of Health Behavior

Among the health behavior theories and models that currently predominate in the field of health promotion and communication are the Health Belief Model, the Communication/Persuasion Model, the Theory of Reasoned Action, the Transtheoretical Model, the Precede/Proceed model, the Diffusions of Innovations model, social learning theory, and applied behavior analysis. The first section of this chapter briefly describes leading health behavior theories and models, in order to put applied behavior analysis in context. The second section describes those principles of behavior analysis that are relevant to the communication process.

Health Belief Model

The Health Belief Model (Rosenstock, 1974, 1977) is closely identified with the field of health education. It holds that health behavior is a function of both knowledge and attitudes. Specifically, this model emphasizes that one's perception of vulnerability to an illness and of the efficacy of treatment will influence one's decisions about health behaviors.

According to the Health Belief Model (Becker, 1974, 1979), behavior is determined by whether individuals (1) believe that they are susceptible to a particular health problem; (2) regard this problem as serious; (3) are convinced that treatment or prevention activities are effective and (4) at the same time inexpensive; and (5) receive a prompt to take health action. For example, a woman may begin to use contraceptives if (1) she already has several children yet knows she has many potential childbearing years ahead of her; (2) sees that her neighbors' health and economic status have been hurt because they have too many children; (3) has heard that a particular contraceptive technique is 95 percent effective and (4) at the same time safe and inexpensive; and (5) was prompted by her health worker to begin taking contraceptives.

Although the various elements of the Health Belief Model have been shown to be statistically related to health behavior, the model has a variety of weaknesses as well. First, health beliefs compete with a person's other beliefs and attitudes, which also may influence behavior. Second, decades of social psychological research have shown that belief formation may actually *follow* rather than precede behavior change. As with other cognitively oriented models, the actual mental processes relative to health belief components may be much more difficult to measure than the behaviors to which they are supposedly causally related. For these and other reasons, other theories of health behavior have attracted increased attention in the past two decades.

Communication/Persuasion Model

The Communication/Persuasion Model (McGuire, 1964) emphasizes that communication can be used to change health attitudes and behaviors, which are directly linked in the same causal chain. The effectiveness of a given communication effort will depend on various inputs (or stimuli) and outputs (or responses to the stimuli). According to this model, changes in knowledge and attitudes are preconditions for health and other behavioral changes. Input variables include the source of a message, the message itself, the channel by which it is sent, receiver characteristics, and destination. Output variables refer to changes in specific cognitive factors, such as knowledge, attitudes, and decision making, as well as observable behaviors.

Theory of Reasoned Action

Also closely identified with health communication is the Theory of Reasoned Action (Fishbein & Ajzen, 1975, 1980), which emphasizes the role of personal intention in determining whether a behavior will occur. The theory implies that behavior generally follows intention and will not occur without it. People's intentions are also influenced by other attitudes toward the behavior such as whether they feel the behavior is important. The theory also emphasizes the "normative" beliefs people may have; that is, what they think other people—in particular, influential people such as peers—would do in a similar situation.

Transtheoretical Model

The Transtheoretical (or "Stages of Change") Model, as suggested by its name, attempts to explain and measure health behavior independent of specific theoretical trappings. Prochaska (1979) and his colleagues initially attempted to describe the process that alcoholics go through when giving up drinking, and later the process of smoking cessation. This research identified four independent stages: precontemplation, contemplation, action, and maintenance.

"Precontemplation" refers to the stage when the person does not even think about the behavior, let alone whether to change it. In the "contemplation" stage, the individual actually considers changing the behavior but is not quite ready to take the plunge. "Action" refers to that aspect of the sequence where the behavior change is initiated, whereas "maintenance" is the longer-term solidification of that change. During either action or maintenance, "relapse" can occur, whereby the individual reverts to the pattern of behavior that preceded the "action" stage.

The stages stipulated in the Transtheoretical Model can be applied to the case of domestic hygiene. Initially, a homemaker—perhaps because she lacks the requisite knowledge or training—does not even consider covering food, boiling water, or keeping a kitchen clean. After hearing a radio spot explaining the rudiments of germ theory and seeing a neighbor scrub down her domicile, she begins to contemplate taking action toward a higher level of hygiene. She gets information from the neighbor and her local health worker and at last begins the behavior change process. After a period of time, she covers food, boils drinking water, and keeps the kitchen environment clean as a matter of her daily routine.

Although its originators consider this model theory-free, they also note that individuals weigh the pros and cons of behavior change before progressing from one stage to the next. For example, the abovementioned homemaker may balance the pros of a healthier life-style and more aesthetic environment against the cons of having less time to care for her children and spending part of her limited household revenues for disinfectant. When this "decisional balance" tips in favor of hygiene, she will move to (or toward) the action stage. In this fashion, the Transtheoretical Model parallels other rational or decision-making and economic theories, especially in its reliance on cognitive processes to explain behavioral change. An exciting recent development in research generated by this model is the attempt to match intervention approaches to the particular stage of change that a target audience is in. For example, imparting information may be the most effective approach to influencing precontemplators, whereas skills training and cues work best for moving contemplators to action, and reinforcement keeps maintainers from relapsing. The Transtheoretical Model is currently the subject of many public health research efforts in both chronic and infectious disease control.

Precede/Proceed Model

Over a decade ago, Lawrence Green and his colleagues developed the now famous Precede/Proceed model for planning health education programs (Green, Kreuter, Deeds, & Partridge, 1980; Green & Kreuter, 1991). Although based in the Health Belief Model and other conceptual systems, Precede is a true "model," meant for pragmatic efforts to change health behavior rather than for theory development. Green and his colleagues analyze a community's health needs by specifying five different "diagnoses": social, epidemiological, behavioral, educational, and administrative/policy. With this model, the health planner avoids the "victim blaming" that often accompanies individually focused needs assessment and evaluation and, instead, keeps the focus on the community level. Nevertheless, the behavioral and educational diagnoses both stress behavior-environment relationships.

Consistent with a behavioral perspective, the educational diagnosis phase of Precede emphasizes "predisposing," "enabling," and "reinforcing" factors. The former two relate to antecedents of a behavior and the skills necessary for its performance, whereas reinforcing factors are synonymous with the term *consequences* used in behavior analysis.

Diffusion of Innovations

The Diffusion of Innovations model (Rogers & Shoemaker, 1971; Rogers, 1973) emphasizes the role of change agents in the social environment, thus taking the focus somewhat away from the ultimate target individual. The relative, neighbor, health worker, or other change agent may help produce behavior change in a variety of ways—for example, by developing a need for change, establishing the necessary interpersonal relationship, identifying the problem and its causes, specifying goals and potential solutions, motivating someone to attempt and maintain action, and terminating the change relationship.

Social Learning Theory

Social learning theory stresses the triadic relationship among "person" (that is, one's cognitive processes), behavior, and environment through a "reciprocal determinism" (or "reciprocal causality") process (Bandura, 1977; Rotter, 1954). In other words, whereas the environment largely determines or causes behavior, the individual uses cognitive processes to interpret both the environment and his or her behavior, and also behaves in ways to change the environment and meet with more favorable behavioral outcomes. Thus, social learning theory bridges the gap between the cognitively oriented rational-decision-making models and behavioral theory emphasized in this book.

Social learning theory views behavior as a function of a person's "self-efficacy" (self-confidence) and outcome expectations. A person becomes confident about his or her ability as a result of past experience with a behavior or observation of others as they successfully performed the behavior. The assumption is that expectations of positive or negative outcomes also will depend on personal or vicarious experiences.

Vicarious (observational) learning is a central theme of social learning theory. Simply stated, when we see someone else (a "model") perform a behavior, our ability to "reproduce" that behavior is enhanced. Bandura divides vicarious learning into four steps: (1) attention to the model, (2) retention of what was observed, (3) reproduction of the behavior, and (4) reinforcement of the behavior. Reinforcement can be vicarious when the learner sees the model meeting with a positive outcome for his or her behavior. Additionally, "learners" may reinforce themselves or may receive reinforcement from others.

The concepts highlighted in social learning theory are depicted in Figure 2.1. Through the process of self-efficacy assessment, the person judges his or her own level of skills and responds to the question "Can I do it, and how well?" Through recollection of outcomes experienced personally or by others, the person responds to the question "Will it pay off?" If the person answers "yes" to both questions, the behavior is likely to occur. Actual reinforce-

Figure 2.1. Interactive Influences on Behavior as Viewed by Social Learning Theorists.

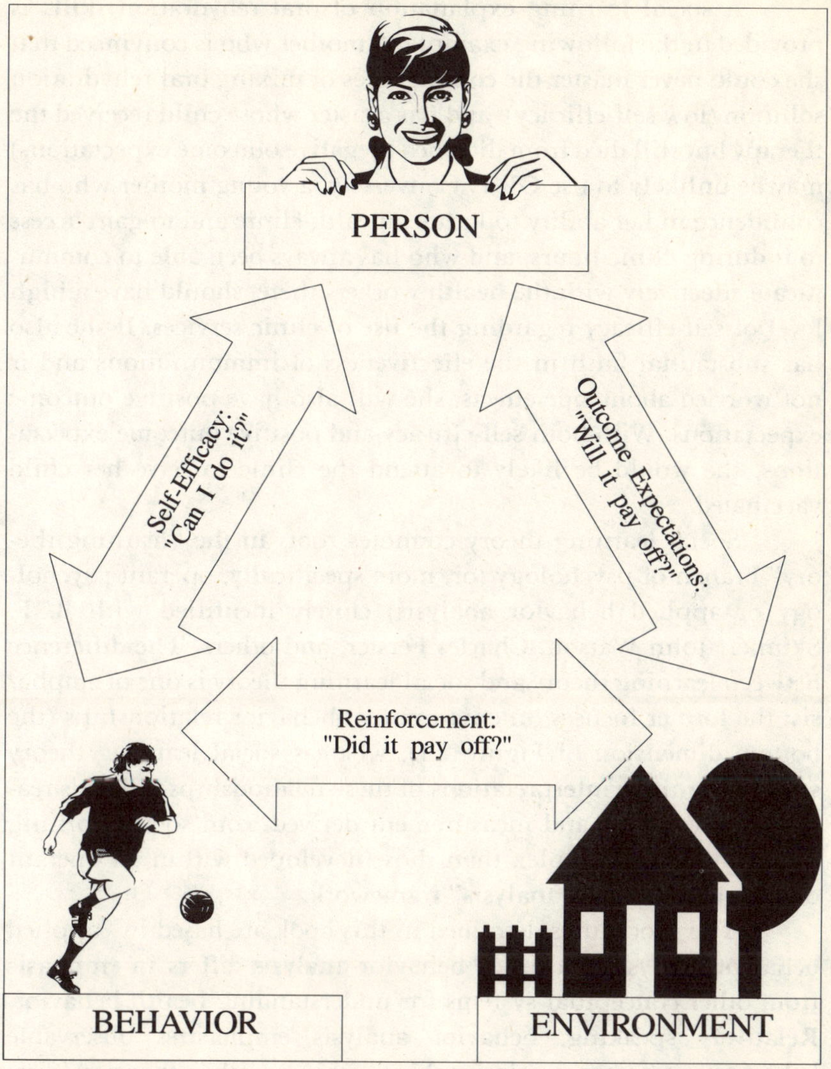

ment—the environmental "reaction" to the behavior—will then help determine whether the behavior will occur again in the future.

A social learning explanation of oral rehydration skills is provided in the following example. A mother who is convinced that she could never master the complexities of mixing oral rehydration solution (low self-efficacy), and has a sister whose child received the therapy but still died from diarrhea (negative outcome expectations) may be unlikely to use ORT. Conversely, a young mother who has confidence in her ability to locate a health clinic and to gain access to it during clinic hours, and who has always been able to communicate effectively with the health workers there, should have a high level of self-efficacy regarding the use of clinic services. If she also has substantial faith in the effectiveness of immunizations and is not worried about side effects, she will also have positive outcome expectations. With both self-efficacy and positive outcome expectations, she would be likely to attend the clinic to have her child vaccinated.

Social learning theory connotes roots in the "learning theory" branch of psychology (or, more specifically, operant psychology or applied behavior analysis) closely identified with B. F. Skinner, John Watson, Charles Ferster, and others. The difference between learning theory and social learning theory is one of emphasis: the former focuses on environment-behavior relationships (the bottom dimension of Figure 2.1), whereas social learning theory stresses cognitive interpretations of these relationships. For this reason, interventions and measurement derived from social learning theory are more complex than those developed within an operant or "applied behavior analysis" framework.

The procedures described in this book are based in "applied behavior analysis." Applied behavior analysis differs in emphasis from other conceptual systems for understanding health behavior. Relatively speaking, behavior analysis emphasizes observable behavior-consequence relationships, whereas other theories focus more on cognitions and antecedent-behavior relationships. Nevertheless, many elements of our presentation (for example, the use of modeling in Chapter Five) are directly related to other health behavior theories and models, especially social learning theory. Therefore, readers already well versed in theory will notice an occasional blending of these two complementary perspectives.

Applied Behavior Analysis: Basic Terms

We now turn to a discussion of the basics, or ABCs, of applied behavior analysis.

Antecedents

Antecedents are environmental events that set the stage for or trigger behavior (Holland & Skinner, 1961; Sulzer-Azaroff & Mayer, 1977; Bandura, 1977; Miller, 1980). A crying baby reminds the mother to feed him; the phone rings and you answer it. Antecedents that reliably signal the time for a behavior increase the likelihood that the behavior will occur at an appropriate time and place. Radio spots that remind parents to take their children to the clinic on immunization day and skills-training programs that prepare people to carry out a health practice function as antecedents for those behaviors.

Many behaviors are automatically triggered by environmental events that we call naturally occurring antecedents. For example, the onset of diarrhea or fever is a natural antecedent that triggers a set of behaviors (either appropriate or inappropriate) in the mother and the health worker. On the other hand, many important health behaviors have no naturally occurring antecedents to trigger them. In those cases, communicators might introduce reminders to trigger the target behavior. These we will call "planned antecedents." For example, immunization is a preventive behavior with no naturally occurring antecedents; there are no signs in a child that indicate she is ready for a vaccination. The communication program might, therefore, introduce antecedents by teaching mothers the immunization schedule, broadcasting spot reminders, or placing posters with the immunization schedule in visible places.

Consequences

Consequences are environmental events that follow a behavior and either strengthen, weaken, or stop it (Holland & Skinner, 1961;

Miller, 1980). Generally, people tend to repeat behaviors that lead to positive results (positive consequences) and to avoid behaviors that produce negative results. The word reinforcement refers to events that strengthen behavior.

Positive reinforcement is a pleasant, agreeable event that follows a behavior: a child's health improves after treatment; a clinic worker praises a mother whose child is growing well; a trainee receives a diploma for mastering skills during training. This type of reinforcement *strengthens the behavior or increases the likelihood that it will occur again* (Baer, Wolf, & Risley, 1968; Miller, 1980).

Negative reinforcement is an ongoing unpleasant, disagreeable event (or a perception of an event); it also strengthens behavior, since a person will tend to repeat a behavior that stops the unpleasant event. For example, more and more people are using condoms, in spite of the inconvenience and negative social sanctions, to relieve their fear of contracting AIDS. Lowering their fear is what reinforces condom usage. People may try various behaviors to make a negative event stop happening: to stop an infant from crying, a mother will change the diaper, comfort the baby, and feed it. The behavior that finally stops the event will most likely be tried in the future (Rimm & Masters, 1979; Karoly & Harris, 1986).

Punishment is a negative consequence that suppresses or weakens behavior. Parents spank their children to make them stop an undesired behavior. A mother who is scolded for being late for an immunization is likely not to return to the clinic. These events act as punishment because the behavior they follow is unlikely to occur again (Sandler, 1986).

Health communicators primarily use positive reinforcement in designing program events to support behavior. Nevertheless, since many people act to avoid punishment (a health worker fills out reports to avoid criticism from the supervisor) or to terminate a negative reinforcement (a mother breast-feeds to stop her infant from crying), communicators need to understand all types of consequences when assessing what is currently maintaining health practices in a community.

The following are other characteristics of consequences important to health communication (see Rimm & Masters, 1979; Miller, 1980):

1. *A consequence that immediately follows a behavior is far more powerful in influencing behavior than one that occurs after a time delay.* The immediate pleasant sensation of smoking a cigarette reinforces this unhealthy habit despite the long-term negative health consequences it causes.
2. *The more salient, relevant, important, or meaningful a consequence is to the individual, the more powerful is its influence on that individual's behavior.* In Nigeria, nutritionists believed that the most important consequence of introducing an enriched weaning food to rural mothers was appropriate growth in their children, and they tried to convince mothers to use it for that reason. Mothers who finally tried the new weaning food became sold on it largely because their children were less cranky and clinging during weaning months. That consequence was far more relevant to their daily life than nutritional benefits were.
3. *A concrete consequence is more powerful than an abstract one.* The concrete consequence of having to walk to the clinic and wait in a crowded room for immunization is often more powerful than the abstract benefit of preventing childhood diseases.
4. *Once a behavior is learned, pleasant consequences need not follow every occurrence of the behavior to maintain it.* For example, during training, health workers need frequent feedback and encouragement from the instructor. Once they have learned to perform the skill correctly, periodic observation and feedback from the supervisor will maintain their performance.

Consequences that occur automatically after a behavior is performed—for instance, a mother gives chloroquine and the child's fever is reduced—are called naturally occurring consequences. Unfortunately, since many of the health practices that communicators are promoting are preventive in nature, they usually produce no immediate, positive, concrete, or salient natural consequences. In this case, a program needs to introduce "planned consequences" to support the desired behavior until naturally occurring ones are observed. Planned consequences can be material rewards such as certificates, lottery prizes, T-shirts, and bars of soap. However, social reinforcement—such as recognition from family members, community leaders, and supervisors or constructive feedback on one's performance—is often more powerful than material rewards.

If a program must introduce consequences, those consequences should be culturally relevant and meaningful to the target audience. What a physician or a communication planner consider an important consequence may not necessarily be important to a mother. As with other programmatic decisions, selection of consequences used in a communication program should be based on research with the target audience. For example, a communication program in Indonesia was asked to improve the low performance rate of village health workers. The communicators conducted a small survey, asking the workers what would make their jobs more rewarding. Various options were suggested, such as T-shirts and badges or attention from supervisors (since the workers were volunteers, payment was not an option). The research revealed that the workers preferred some form of recognition from their own community: village leaders, neighbors, and local groups. Recognition from them was far more meaningful (a more salient consequence) than material rewards or work-related advantages.

Behavior

Having reviewed antecedents and consequences, we also need to look closely at the target behavior itself, because the characteristics of that behavior have important implications for communication strategies (Nelson & Hayes, 1981). Target behavior, such as giving a vitamin A capsule to a child or exclusively breast-feeding a newborn, is the behavioral goal of a health communication program. When looking at a target behavior, communicators consider whether:

The target behavior exists, but not in sufficient frequency. For example, parents seek some but not all immunizations in the series.

The target behavior exists, but not in sufficient duration. Parents give chloroquine only until the fever is reduced and not for the number of days required.

The target behavior exists, but not in the form desired. Mothers breast-feed, but they introduce other foods and liquids too early.

The target behavior exists, but not at the right time. Mothers seek medical care when a child has a head cold rather than when the child shows signs of pneumonia.

The target behavior does not exist at all. Some women do not come to health centers for prenatal care and tetanus vaccinations.

A competing behavior exists. A competing behavior is one that, when practiced, interferes with another behavior. For example, bottle feeding competes with breast feeding. In attempting to discourage an unhealthy practice, a communicator could promote a new, healthy behavior that competes with the existing practice and might eventually replace it. Many programs promote oral rehydration salts (ORS) and available fluids, rather than explicitly discouraging other treatments for diarrhea.

The target behavior is complex. Desirable health practices are frequently more complex than they may at first glance appear to be. In such instances, communicators may break the target behavior into discrete steps, in order to understand what is demanded of those who are to practice it and to help them learn the behavior more readily. Understanding the complexity of behavior helps communicators appropriately select messages, plan strategies, and design training. By recognizing the complexity of mixing and administering ORS, for example, Honduran communicators were able to design a program that successfully taught this complex set of behaviors in small, manageable steps.

The A-B-C Chain

The relationship between environmental events and behavior is often called the A-B-C chain *(antecedent-behavior-consequence).* This relationship has several implications for health communication.

Antecedent or Consequence? The same event might function sometimes as an antecedent and at other times as a consequence, depending on how it influences behavior. For example, a radio spot can function as an antecedent by reminding mothers to bring their children in for immunizations, but it could also be used as a consequence by complimenting the community for achieving a high coverage rate. In fact, consequences for a behavior may serve as part of the antecedent when that behavior is repeated. Some health campaigns have used diplomas for reinforcing compliance with a medical regimen—for example, the completion of an immunization series. The diploma serves not only as a reinforcer (C_1) for the first visit to the clinic (B_1) but also as a prompt (A_2) to revisit the clinic (B_2) for a second or third booster immunization. This prompt may be especially effective if the diploma is attractive and is displayed on the wall of the home or other visible location. This two-stage sequence is represented in Figure 2.2.

The Power of Consequences. Applied behavior analysts generally agree that consequences exert more influence over the continued occurrence of the behavior than do antecedents (Miller, 1980). A communicator who wants to achieve lasting behavior change would focus on what follows desired behavior and would design strategies to create a favorable set of consequences for those behaviors. These are called consequence strategies. This approach is different from programs that focus primarily on antecedents. Strategies that focus on raising awareness, increasing knowledge, using audiovisual aids, and training are called antecedent strategies. If these interventions are used alone, and without regard to the consequences following a behavior, they are less likely to lead to the adoption of practices.

Linkages in the A-B-C Chain. The most powerful communication programs are those that strengthen the linkages between the antecedent, the occurrence of the behavior, and its consequences. Besides triggering behavior though reminders and added information, antecedent strategies can also strengthen the association between consequences and the target behavior.

Figure 2.2. Antecedents and Consequences of Behavior.

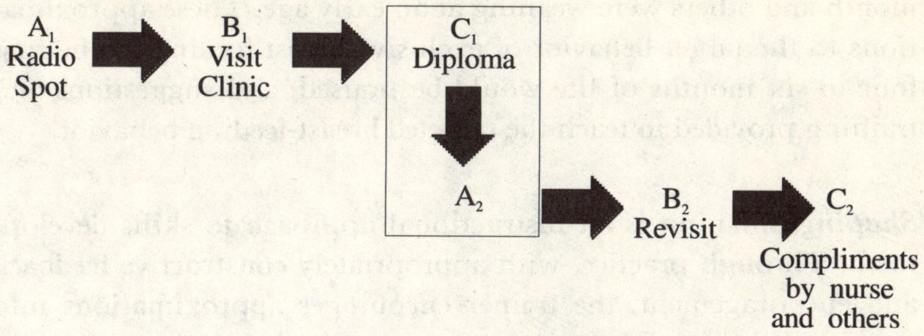

- Such strategies could "market the consequence." For example, radio spots promoting the desirability of immunizations could teach mothers to take pride in a completed immunization card.
- The strategies could signal the availability of pleasant consequences—for example, by promoting a new weaning food as a way to achieve weight gain in an infant.
- They also could teach others how to reinforce behavior. For example, health workers could be trained to praise mothers for correctly mixing ORS or administering it when their children last had diarrhea.

Other Useful Concepts

The following are additional behavioral concepts that will be used throughout this book (see Holland & Skinner, 1961; Rimm & Masters, 1979; Sulzer-Azaroff & Mayer, 1977; Miller, 1980).

Approximations. Frequently, target behaviors are already being practiced in some form. These are called approximations because they are similar to the target behavior, but they are not performed correctly or at the right time, duration, or frequency. An effective communication strategy builds on these approximations by reinforcing those aspects of the behavior that people are doing well and correcting what they need to change. For example, a regional survey showed that most mothers were breast-feeding their infants. It also showed, however, that some were introducing liquids in the first month and others were weaning at an early age. These approximations to the target behavior of exclusive breast feeding in the first four to six months of life would be praised, and suggestions and training provided to teach the targeted breast-feeding behavior.

Shaping. Shaping is an instructional approach to skills development. Through practice, with appropriately constructive feedback and encouragement, the trainer encourages approximations into the ideal behavior. The primary purpose of role play in skills training is to shape approximations to desired behaviors through systematic and repeated practice and feedback.

Fading. Fading is the gradual withdrawal of artificially introduced antecedents or consequences. When a program must introduce prompts or rewards to encourage new behavior, the program should also be designed so that slowly, over time, those elements will be withdrawn as more naturally occurring antecedents or consequences begin to take place. Successful fading to naturally occurring events is critical in maintaining behavior change over time.

Skills Versus Performance Deficit. A person may be unable to perform a target behavior because he or she lacks specific information, tools, or abilities (that is, because of a skills deficit). After acquiring the necessary skills, the person still may perform the behavior incorrectly because conditions in the environment are not supportive of repeated correct behavior (that is, because of a performance deficit). For example, a health worker may have learned how to give a health talk after receiving months of training; however, working with no supervision in a crowded, understaffed clinic, and with sporadic pay, she may infrequently use the skills she learned and enjoys doing. During planning, communicators need to determine to what extent skills and performance deficits are contributing to the absence of the target behavior and select and design appropriate communication.

Learning Conditions Versus Maintenance Conditions. Conditions that produce the best learning (for example, breaking complex behavior into simple steps and providing extra reinforcers and immediate, constructive, and rewarding feedback) are not necessarily required to maintain a learned behavior. Communication programs designed for maintaining target behavior will use different strategies from those effective in initiating and teaching new behaviors.

Characteristics of Programs Applying Behavior Analysis

Public health communication programs that apply the principles derived from behavior analysis will have several characteristics in common.

- *They will focus on observable behaviors.* Communication strategies introduce and maintain changes in behavior, rather than increasing knowledge or improving attitudes about health practices. Direct observation of behavior is, therefore, an important research, information-gathering, and evaluation technique throughout the communication process.
- *They will design either for behavior change or for behavior maintenance.* Program design for initiation of behavior may be different from program design for behavior maintenance. For example, media messages for promoting initiation of behaviors may emphasize future benefits to be gained and the specific skills involved. Messages helping to maintain a learned behavior will congratulate people for making the change and encourage them to reach out to "late adapters."
- *They will shift the emphasis of communication strategies from antecedents to consequences.* Program activities are designed to focus on creating an environment to support desired behaviors. In many cases, subgroups of the target audience will already be using the desired behavior. When these people are given reinforcement, they will be more likely to maintain the behavior; at the same time, "later adapters" will be better able to see its benefits.
- *They will accommodate the complexity of desired health practices in program design.* Communicators will choose among

complex health behaviors those that are feasible for the target audience to perform. In teaching a complex health behavior, communicators break it down into sequential steps to enhance learning.

Summary

Social learning theory; the Theory of Reasoned Action; and the Health Belief, Transtheoretical, and Precede/Proceed models all look at person-environment-behavior interactions in explaining or planning for health behavior change. Behavior analysis departs from these conceptual systems in its emphasis on observable behavior and on behavior-consequence relationships. Immediate and salient positive reinforcement can be an effective tool for changing health behavior, particularly if the lack of behavior is the result of performance rather than skills deficits. In general health communicators need to consider antecedents and consequences when designing communication strategies for all participants in the health process: mothers, family members, health care providers, supervisors, community leaders, policy makers, and donors.

3

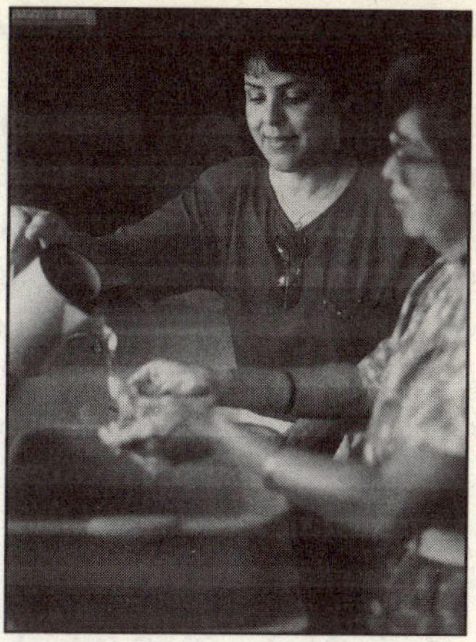

Assessing Behavior

Assessment is the first stage of the communication process. During this stage, communicators gather information to plan communication strategies based on the needs, cultural context, and practices of the target audience. They begin a dialogue with the community through research with representatives of the target audience, thereby shifting the focus from technical issues to the actions that people need to take to respond to the health problem (Rasmuson, Seidel, Smith, & Booth, 1988; Smith, 1989; Smith & Furst, 1986).

To plan a behaviorally focused communication program, communicators need to define the "ideal behavior"; that is, during assessment, communicators need to provide a thorough description of the medically prescribed steps necessary to have maximum impact on the health problem (Kanfer & Saslow, 1969). They also need to collect information about the target audience's existing health practices and the antecedents and consequences influencing these practices (see Sulzer-Azaroff & Mayer, 1977). This information will be used during planning to select target behaviors, to design strategies, and to determine how to use communication channels. In addition, communicators need information about the target audience's media usage, institutional support, and interpersonal communication channels (Novelli, 1990; Israel, Foote, & Tognetti, 1987; Kendall, Foote, & Martorell, 1983). These areas are beyond the scope of this book. A list of suggested supplemental readings for this chapter appears at the end of this book.

During assessment, the communicator seeks answers to three questions related to existing practices of the target audience and the antecedents and consequences that might influence them.

- What behaviors related to the health problem is the target audience presently performing? Which ones are approximations to ideal behaviors? Which ones compete with desired behaviors?
- Is the absence of desired behaviors due to a skills deficit (lack of skills necessary to perform the behavior) or to a performance deficit (existing conditions and resources do not support the behavior)?
- What consequences exist for both desired and competing behaviors? If target behaviors produce few, if any, naturally occurring positive consequences, what antecedent and consequence strategies could the communication program develop to strengthen target behaviors?

Answers to these questions help to shift the communicator's focus from technical issues to behavioral ones.

Steps in Conducting Behavioral Assessment

Behavioral assessment involves analyzing the health practice and defining the ideal behavior, reviewing secondary research, and conducting formative research. The result will be the information necessary to plan for a behaviorally focused communication program.

Step 1: Analyze the Health Practice and Define the "Ideal Behavior"

One of the principal questions to be answered during the planning process is "What does the target audience need to *do* in order to achieve an effective health practice?" What behaviors will the communication program need to introduce, teach, and support? Although health practices frequently appear simple, they actually involve a complex set of decisions and actions that communicators must thoroughly understand before they can plan an effective communication program. The assessment process begins, therefore, with a detailed analysis of the health practice and a definition of the "ideal behavior": a list of discrete, sequential steps of the antecedents, behaviors, and consequences of the health practice in its medically prescribed, ideal form (Sulzer-Azaroff & Mayer, 1977; Hersen & Bellack, 1981).

At this step, the communicator needs to form an interdisciplinary team to guide him through the multiple decisions that will be made during assessment and planning. The team would be composed of a combination of medical specialists (epidemiologist, maternal and child health specialist, disease specific specialist, nutritionist), communicators (health educator, social marketer, mass media specialist), and social scientists (behavioral psychologist, anthropologist, operations researcher). The composition of this team may change as needs evolve. (See Chapter Six for suggested team composition at the monitoring phase.)

It is not always easy to define the ideal behavior. Several common issues usually provoke discussion and disagreement among experts. First, the process of focusing on behavior and breaking it down into steps reveals how complicated the behavior really is. Second, there may be several ways to perform a behavior "ideally," and these different ways may be equally correct. For example, in breast feeding, the "ideal" way for a mother to hold and support a child depends on the age of the infant and on the mother's position (whether she is sitting or lying down). Third, experts frequently disagree about which behaviors are really necessary to have health impact, especially in those areas where no data exist to support one behavior over another. In their attempts to define ideal hand-washing behavior, for example, the group of experts designing communication strategies had lengthy discussions concerning how many times the hands should be rubbed together, whether the mother should clean under her fingernails, and whether each finger should be scrubbed separately. Finally, technical experts may disagree on what the ideal behavior should look like; technical norms are constantly changing as new data emerge. Discussions and disagreements between team members are natural and healthy. Team members should accept disagreement as part of the process and not let it deter them from looking closely at the behaviors they wish to change. Team members will have another opportunity to review the list of ideal behaviors after they have observed what people are actually doing.

In compiling the list, the team should consider *antecedents*—enabling knowledge and skills and physical materials necessary to perform the behavior; *behavior*—the specific sequential steps required to perform the behavior correctly; and *consequences*—both natural consequences that result when the behavior is performed and ideas for planned consequences that could be temporarily introduced. During the process, communicators should encourage the creativity of this interdisciplinary team by asking its members to consider the various alternatives in each category. Focused research will provide information about the target audience to fill in the gaps in the team's analysis.

Exhibit 3.1 is an example of the "ideal behavior" for oral rehydration therapy (ORT) as developed by the Honduras Diarrheal Disease Control Program.

Exhibit 3.1. Ideal Behavior for ORT: Honduras Diarrheal Disease Control Program.

TREATMENT BEHAVIORS CONSIDERED

Diagnosis

1. Recognize that the child's stool is abnormal.
2. Confirm that the following pre-acute symptoms are present:

   watery stool
   listlessness
   loss of appetite
   more than three stools in a day

3. Confirm that the following acute symptoms are present:

   sunken eyes
   dry skin/mouth
   diarrhea and vomiting

4. Confirm the following decision patterns:

   If 2 is no and 3 is no, take action.
   If 2 is yes and 3 is no, use home-based ORT.
   If 2 is yes and 3 is yes, go to hospital/clinic.

Acceptance

5. Identify ORT packet as medicine for dehydration—not diarrhea.
6. Identify packet as capable of restoring appetite and activity.
7. Identify packet as incapable of reducing the number of watery stools.
8. Identify packet as capable of replacing essential fluids.
9. Identify rehydration medicine as better than purge, starvation, and folk remedies.

Exhibit 3.1. Ideal Behavior for ORT: Honduras Diarrheal Disease Control Program, Cont'd.

10. Identify the cost of the ORT packet in local currency.
11. State why expenditure and effort are worth it.

Procurement

12. Name packet.
13. Identify packet visually.
14. Identify location(s) where packet can be obtained.
15. State that two packets should be purchased each time.
16. State how they will obtain packet.

Mixing

17. Identify a one-liter vessel.
18. State that the vessel must be washed and free from foreign matter.
19. Fill one liter container to the top with cleanest available water.
20. Open the packet without spilling.
21. Add the contents of one packet with minimal spillage.
22. Add nothing else to solution.
23. Stir or shake.
24. Identify dissolved solution.
25. State that the mixture should NOT be boiled.

Administration

26. Use a small spoon to give the entire liter in small amounts.
27. Administer small amounts continuously through waking hours.
28. Continue to breast-feed while rehydrating.
29. If child vomits, allow him or her to rest for a few minutes and start to give small amounts again slowly.
30. Feed child weaning foods (agua de arroz, ploedas atoles) as soon as appetite returns.
31. Never withhold food.
32. If diarrhea continues after first day, mix and give new solution for one more day, or until after diarrhea stops.

Seeking Medical Help

33. If diarrhea continues for more than two days, seek medical help.
34. If vomiting occurs five or more times a day, seek medical help.
35. Give child ORT solution during trip to clinic if possible.

Recovery Nutrition

36. Feed soft-boiled eggs every day for ten days after appetite returns.
37. After appetite returns, offer more food than usual.
38. Offer supplementary food for as many days as child had diarrhea.

Source: Rasmuson, Seidel, Smith, & Booth, 1988, pp. 24–26. Reprinted with permission.

As can be observed, the health practice of diarrhea treatment was divided into seven main categories of behaviors: diagnosis, acceptance, procurement, mixing, administration, seeking medical help, and recovery nutrition. Within a specific behavioral category were discrete steps necessary to carry out the behavior. Some of the behavioral steps within a category were initially listed as several alternatives, and then focus-group discussions were used to explore these alternatives with the target audience and to choose the one to be promoted by the program. For example, three alternative steps were considered under the category "Recovery Nutrition": feed soft-boiled eggs every day for ten days after appetite returns; after appetite returns, offer more food than usual; and offer supplementary food for as many days as the child had diarrhea. This research indicated that rural women regarded the third suggested step (offering supplementary food for as many days as the child had diarrhea) as the most feasible behavior to adopt. This behavior was then selected as the target for the communication program.

Case Study: Defining the Ideal Behavior in a Guatemalan Water and Sanitation Program

In Guatemala, the Nutrition Institute for Central America and Panama (INCAP) received funding from the World Health Organization to implement a communication program designed to lower diarrheal morbidity through increased use of a newly installed community water system. An interdisciplinary team—made up of an epidemiologist, a physician, two health communicators, a regional health trainer, and an anthropologist—met to define the ideal behavior and areas of formative research to be conducted during the assessment stage.

After selecting "mother's hand washing" as the target health practice for the program, the interdisciplinary team began to define the "ideal behavior"—the list of discrete, sequential steps they felt were necessary to perform this practice correctly. The anthropologist guided team members in washing their hands, using materials generally found in the home (water taken from a large jug, a small bowl to rinse the hands, and so on). Team members timed the duration of each hand-washing performance and measured the amount of water used. They found that what had originally appeared to be a relatively simple behavior actually needed forty-six steps to perform correctly. Nine items related to the times when the mother should wash her hands: after using the latrine, after changing a dirty diaper, before preparing food, before eating, before giving food to the infant, upon entering the home, before going to bed, and before touching the cooking or drinking water. Correct hand washing required an average of 600 cc of water. Their observations of how long it took to wash hands indicated that an average of two minutes was required. The team discovered that if a mother performed "correct hand washing," she would actually spend almost an hour a day washing her hands! The amount of water needed required the mother to carry an additional jug of water to her home each day, just for her own correct hand washing.

This exercise demonstrated that hand washing in its ideal form has a very high cost to the mother, in both time and water expended. The team members realized this cost needed to be lowered if hand washing was to be widely practiced. They decided to use formative research to test the Tippy-Tap, a simple hand-washing device originally developed in Africa, which reduces the amount of water needed for hand washing. Could this attractive new technology motivate people to engage in this health practice? Unfortunately, fifty-four steps were identified for the fabrication, installation, and maintenance of the Tippy-Tap. The team decided to use formative research to understand how the communication strategy could engage other family members to perform some of the behavioral steps needed to make, install, and maintain this device (E. Hurtado, Institute for Central America and Panama, personal communication, 1992).

Defining the ideal behavior was critical to this interdisciplinary team in understanding the complexity and cost of the health practice and identifying areas of research to be conducted during the assessment stage. The communication strategy that was developed as a result of this research will be discussed in Chapter Four.

Step 2: Review Secondary Research

Frequently, research studies have been conducted on current behaviors relative to the health practice and the environment in which it functions; so communicators need only conduct small, focused studies to fill in the gaps. Before designing additional research, communicators should identify and review existing data from ongoing projects, donor reports, and local training institutions. These data might include ethnographies, prevalence surveys, and other studies of knowledge, attitudes, and practices (KAP studies) (Pelto, 1991). Although these documents are not always easy to track down, they can save valuable time and resources in the long run. Some of the places to find existing research in a country include the USAID mission (its health, population, and nutrition offices), UNICEF and WHO country offices, the Ministry of Health and other ministries, nongovernmental organizations, medical and public health schools, hospitals, and the departments of social sciences and anthropology at local universities.

Step 3: Conduct Formative Research

Formative research is research conducted for the purpose of developing ("forming") communication strategies (Debus, 1988). Both quantitative and qualitative methods are used to provide data for planning communication strategies in general and for designing health messages in particular. The data are collected from the people who perform the health practice or from the people who support the practice. For example, a survey may need to include questions about where mothers seek help and information when their children have acute respiratory infections (ARI), or an observational study may be done to see what consequences follow the performance of a target behavior.

Health communicators can use a variety of research techniques to understand a target audience's knowledge, attitudes, and practices concerning the health problem (Debus, 1988). These techniques are also used to collect information on other people—such as health workers, husbands, and pharmacists—who are important in influencing the target audience's behavior. Some of the most common techniques include:

- Surveys—a quantitative research technique that permits researchers to determine the percent of the population who think or act in a specified way. Surveys may be conducted at a household level with a random or purposive sample. Communicators may also select locations most relevant to their specific target audience. At these locations, such as markets, village wells, and bus depots, they conduct small-sample surveys. These are called central location intercept interviews.
- Focus group discussion—a qualitative research technique in which a moderator leads a small homogeneous group of respondents (six to ten) through a discussion of a selected topic. Focus-group discussions are repeated with other groups of participants (usually two to four groups in all) until no new information is revealed. The moderator uses a prepared list of probing questions to collect information, but at the same time allows discussants to talk freely and spontaneously about the selected health problem. The information gathered cannot be quantified, and generalizations based on the results should be carefully made. Nevertheless, focus groups and other qualitative research techniques can help communicators understand why people think or act as they do.
- In-depth interview—a qualitative research technique consisting of intensive individual interviews with a small number of respondents to explore what people think and say they do about the health topic.
- Ethnomedical study—the use of anthropological techniques to analyze how specific health practices relate to the larger cultural context. These studies require several months and a trained ethnographer, but they provide invaluable information about how cultural beliefs influence health practices.
- Behavior observation. The researcher observes a specific set of behaviors to understand how well, how long, and how frequently they are performed. Data from these observations can be quantified and complement research that relies on verbal report. (Specific types of observation are discussed later in this chapter.)

To plan a behaviorally focused communication program, communicators would need to take the following steps:

1. Use qualitative and quantitative research to explore the consequences of the health practice and to find out what respondents say they know and do about it.

2. Conduct direct observation. A characteristic of behaviorally focused communication is that research tools are designed to measure behavior change throughout the health communication process; the same research techniques and instruments developed during assessment are used again in the design and implementation of training, supervision, monitoring, and evaluation. Communicators can conduct discrete observational studies, or they can add direct observation to other research techniques. For example, in an in-depth interview, a focus group, or a survey, the researcher might ask a mother to mix oral rehydration salts, the behavior being discussed.

Using Qualitative and Quantitative Research to Understand Consequences

Typically, qualitative and quantitative research studies focus on what respondents know and feel about a health problem and what they say they do about it (Eiseman, Patel, & Sena, 1987). Yet improving knowledge, attitudes, and even skills about a specific behavior might not be sufficient to change that behavior if the consequences are working against the change. Communicators can use quantitative and qualitative research to explore specific behavior-consequence relationships in both desired and competing behaviors. In this case, the KAP surveys could be conceptualized as "KAP-C": knowledge-attitude-practices-consequences research. In health communication programs, this distinction can prove to be very important, particularly if the absence of the desired behavior seems to be due to unfavorable consequences rather than to a lack of skills.

When a person is already engaging in the desired behavior—for example, a mother who brings her child to the clinic for all three DPT vaccinations—the communicator can use the research opportunity to ask questions about what types of consequences are maintaining this desired behavior. Questions might include:

"What happened the last time you took your child to be vaccinated at the clinic? How long did you wait? How did the clinic staff treat you?"

"How does your child act after he is vaccinated?"

"What did your husband do or say when you returned from the clinic?"

Communicators can also use qualitative and quantitative research to explore why a person does *not* perform the behavior or practices a competing behavior (see Debus, 1988). Questions related to the consequences to mothers administering an antidiarrheal, rather than ORS, might include:

"What happens to your child when you give an antidiarrheal?"

"How does your mother-in-law react when you give antidiarrheal?"

"What would happen if you didn't give an antidiarrheal and gave ORS instead?"

Including questions about consequences in quantitative and qualitative research will provide communicators with information critical to planning their behaviorally focused communication program, especially if the absence of the behavior is due to a performance deficit.

Using Qualitative and Quantitative Research to Address Specific Behavioral Questions

In general, communicators planning research that will aid in developing communication strategies should first clearly state program objectives in terms of desired behaviors. Then, different kinds of research can be used to identify important aspects of behavior.

Identify and Understand Existing Behavior and Its Consequences. Communicators often have very little existing (empirical) information about the prevailing practice of behaviors relevant to the health problem being addressed. Qualitative and quantitative research opportunities can be used to explore these practices. In Honduras, for example, the Ministry of Health wanted to begin a more aggressive acute respiratory infection (ARI) program, but had very little research data on mothers' current knowledge, attitudes, and practices. In-depth interviews were conducted to assess mothers' skills with respect to home management of acute respiratory infections. Specifically, researchers asked what signs of ARI the mothers attended to, what types of medicines they used, and which of several items (kleenex, Q-tips, or a cloth) mothers preferred to use for clearing nasal passages.

Develop a Detailed List of Steps for Performing the Health Practice. During assessment, communicators analyze the complexity of the desired health practice and break it down into a series of discrete, sequential behaviors. In focus-group discussions or individual interviews, mothers can discuss and demonstrate to researchers crucial behaviors related to the health issue or child survival strategy being investigated. In The Gambia, focus-group participants were asked to mix a water-sugar-salt oral rehydration solution following a prerecorded taped message. The researchers were then able to identify steps in the process that had not been included in the instructions and without which the mothers could not mix the solution correctly (Rasmuson and Booth, 1985).

Identify Effective Consequences. When the absence of the desired behavior is due to a performance deficit, the communication strategy will focus on strengthening consequences to support and maintain the desired health practice. As previously mentioned, quantitative and qualitative research can help communicators determine which consequences are the most culturally appropriate, individually salient, and immediate for the specific target audience. Communicators should not assume that certain reinforcers have universal appeal until research has confirmed this assumption. For example, in most Western cultures, recognition given to an individual for good performance is a powerful, positive consequence for performing target behaviors. Many communicators might therefore assume that individual recognition is a fundamental human motivator. However, in many other cultures, individual recognition is not particularly reinforcing because other social units have much more saliency. In The Gambia, for example, focus-group research revealed that rewards for correct diarrhea treatment should be presented to the entire village, as well as to individual mothers.

Behavior Observation

Direct and systematic observation is most useful when the goal of the communication program is behavior change. By using observational assessment, communicators need not rely on self-report to learn how individuals behave in their daily lives. Rather, communicators have direct evidence of this behavior. They can learn, firsthand, the antecedents and consequences of both current and recommended behaviors; they can understand environmentally imposed reasons why particular practices exist or do not exist. In addition, they can analyze and describe the desired new behavior, understand the complexity of the behavior, and measure performance levels of learned behavior (Holland & Skinner, 1961; Kazdin, 1981).

The direct observation of behavior complements assessment via self-report in several ways. Observing practices directly, whether in the clinic or in the home, provides more valid and more detailed data than relying solely on verbal recall. Although each session is labor intensive, observational research uses small samples, which generally require less time and fewer resources than other research methods. As a result, small observational studies are often used in conjunction with other data-gathering techniques as a validation of survey data or as a way of teasing out elements of a complex set of interactions.

Frequently, communicators do not have the resources or the time to conduct separate observational studies. In this case, they can combine research techniques to complement and corroborate findings. One way is to include structured observation in program research. Focus groups, in-depth interviews, and surveys provide excellent opportunities to conduct behavior observation (Debus, 1988). For example, the researcher can ask mothers to wash their hands and can use a performance observation checklist as a part of a focus-group discussion or an in-depth interview.

Types of Observation

Behavior can be observed in the setting where the behavior occurs—the hospital, clinic, office, or home—or in a simulation. Several types of observation are useful in assessing behaviors.

Performance Observation. Performance observation is conducted when the communicator knows what the ideal health practice is and wants to find out how often the behavioral steps (necessary to perform that practice) are performed or how many are performed at a given time. Sample performance checklists are included as resources at the back of this book.

The health practice is first broken down into a series of measurable steps and compiled into a checklist. The researcher then observes the practice and checks off those steps the person executes. For example, an interdisciplinary team could identify the behavioral steps that health workers need to perform for effective interpersonal communication and compile them into a checklist. By using the checklist while observing a number of health talks, supervisors could assess what content areas and teaching techniques need to be emphasized in future training sessions. Performance observation would also be a useful research technique for understanding the current skill levels of mothers as they prepare and administer ORS. Communication messages could be selected to emphasize those steps mothers were not performing correctly or at all. Exhibit 3.2 is a performance checklist for observing a mother as she prepares prepackaged oral rehydration salts in her home.

Exhibit 3.2. Performance Observation: Mixing Oral Rehydration Solution.

x	Uses a container that measures one liter. *(Asks if this is a liter bottle.)*
x	Washed container so it is free from foreign matter.
	Fills container completely with the cleanest water possible *(only 3/4 full).*
x	Opens ORS packet without spilling contents.
x	Adds the contents of one package, with minimal spillage, to the water.
x	Adds nothing else to the solution. *(Asks if she should).*
	Stirs or shakes the solution until all of the salts are dissolved.
x	Does not heat or boil the mixture.

In this performance observation, the observer asked a mother to mix the oral rehydration salts and checked off each of the steps she performed correctly. The observer also noted (in italics) anything else relevant to mixing the salts; for example, the mother was not exactly sure what a liter measure was and asked whether she should add anything else to the mixture. If other mothers repeat this pattern, communicators will conclude that they need to emphasize these specific steps in their training and media messages.

Performance observation can also help communicators discover to what degree approximations to target behaviors exist. These findings are important for planning a training program or for establishing baseline performance levels before a health communication program is launched. The same performance observation can also be used after an intervention, to assess the impact that training or other program activities have had on performance. This application of performance observation is discussed further in Chapter Five. Performance observation also is a useful monitoring tool and is further described in Chapter Six.

Narrative (ABC) Recording. Narrative recording is particularly useful when communicators are unfamiliar with target behaviors and the environmental events that support or deter them. The researcher simply observes a person engaging in the behavior and writes a narrative describing in sequence what transpires. Unlike open-ended observational recording, these observations are organized into a three-column (A-B-C) chart consisting of the events occurring prior to the behavior (antecedents), the subject's responses (behaviors), and the event that follow the behavior (consequences). Narrative recording allows further specification of the conditions in which the behavior occurs and the possible conditions that might maintain the behavior (Kazdin, 1981; Barlow, Hayes, & Nelson, 1984).

For example, in Honduras, communicators suspected that the reasons why mothers were not completing the immunization series had to do with some aspect of clinic policy and practices. A survey showed that mothers had sufficient knowledge about the need for and timing of the immunization schedule, but they were not taking their children to be immunized. The communicators used narrative recording to learn whether certain interactions between mothers and the clinic health worker might deter or support

Exhibit 3.3. Narrative Observation: Immunizations in a Clinic.

Antecedents	*Behaviors (of Mothers)*	*Consequences*
Clinic empty, nurse filling out paperwork	Mother walks in, looks at nurse	Nurse continues to look down at paperwork, does not look up at mother
Several minutes later, nurse motions to mother to approach the examination station with the baby	Mother approaches examination station, hands nurse the baby to be weighed and vaccinated	Nurse takes baby, baby begins to cry
Nurse places baby on scale	Mother looks on attentively	Nurse records weight in chart without saying anything
Nurse injects baby with injection	Mother cringes	Nurse hands crying baby back to mother; nurse says nothing, spends several minutes on chart work

return visits to the clinic, a behavior critical to completing the immunization series. The narrative observation chart presented as Exhibit 3.3 demonstrates some of their results. As can be seen, the health worker did little to encourage the mother during the immunization session; the mother received few pleasant consequences and some unpleasant ones for her behavior. It could be expected that the mother would feel punished by this experience and be less likely to return to the clinic or recommend the experience to her neighbors. The results of this narrative recording provided a variety of suggestions for improving health worker–patient interactions and thereby enhancing compliance with vaccination schedules.

Frequency Recording. Frequency recording is used when the communicator believes the behavior is occurring, but not in sufficient frequency to be an effective health practice (Miller, 1980). During an observational session, the observer simply counts each occurrence of a particular action (such as hand washing) during a designated time period.

Frequency recording is particularly useful when the frequency of the behavior is critical to health impact—for example, in breast feeding, feeding of weaning foods, and feeding during diarrhea episodes. Communicators might use frequency recording to measure the number of spoonfuls of ORS or food a mother administers in a certain number of hours. In Exhibit 3.4, this technique is used to measure the frequency of interpersonal communication

Exhibit 3.4. Clinic Frequency Observation.

Behavior	*Frequency*
Greets mother	✓✓✓✓✓✓✓
Asks mother about her child	✓✓✓✓✓✓
Asks mother open-ended question	✓✓
Praises mother for what she says or does correctly	✓✓✓
Asks mother closed-ended question	✓✓✓✓✓✓✓✓✓✓✓✓
Demonstrates mixing ORS	✓✓✓✓✓✓✓
Has mother demonstrate mixing ORS	

skills demonstrated by a nurse during a series of clinic visits. During frequency observation, the observer watched a clinic nurse's interaction with seven mothers whose children had diarrhea. The observer simply put a check mark in the "Frequency" column each time the clinic worker performed one of the behaviors on the list. The trainer and supervisors would then be able to see which steps of effective interpersonal communication were already being performed in sufficient frequency (in this case, those steps were greeting a mother, asking a mother about her child, asking a mother closed-ended questions, and demonstrating mixing ORS). During supervisory visits, they would be able to praise the nurse for performing those steps. They would also be able to provide specific training in the steps that the nurse is not presently carrying out in sufficient frequency (in this case, asking open-ended questions, praising a mother for what she does or says correctly, and having mothers demonstrate mixing ORS).

Duration Recording. The communicator uses duration recording when he or she believes the target behavior is occurring, but not in sufficient duration to be effective. The observer measures the length of time a specific action occurs during a designated sample time period. The behavior to be measured must have an easily determined beginning and end, so that the observer can accurately and reliably determine the length of time that the behavior was performed during a predefined observation period (Sulzer-Azaroff & Mayer, 1977). Again, any feeding practice (breast feeding, administering ORS, feeding weaning foods, or feeding during illness to maintain the child's weight) increases in health effectiveness the longer each feeding session lasts. The length of time a mother attempts to administer ORS, breast milk, or other foods becomes a critical measure to be taken through observation.

Exhibit 3.5 is an example of the use of duration observation to help researchers understand how clinic practices influence mothers bringing their children to be immunized. During this duration observation, the observer simply noted the time that individual mothers arrived and left the clinic and then calculated the length of their visit. In this case, duration observation demonstrated that immunization of a child took an average of seventy-one minutes

Exhibit 3.5. Clinic Duration Observation.

	Time Arrived	*Time Left*	*Total Duration*
Mother #1	7:15 a.m.	7:50	35 minutes
Mother #2	7:20 a.m.	8:02	42 minutes
Mother #3	7:23 a.m.	8:20	57 minutes
Mother #4	7:25 a.m.	8:45	78 minutes
Mother #5	7:28 a.m.	9:05	97 minutes
Mother #6	7:28 a.m.	9:25	117 minutes

from the moment mothers arrived at the clinic to the moment they left. This finding helped communicators discover a negative consequence that probably would deter mothers from returning frequently enough to immunize their children completely.

Behavioral Products Observation. The effect of a behavior can be measured by means of behavioral products observation. The observer counts the number of "physical" products or effects of a target behavior—for example, the number of used syringes indicates how many children were immunized on a given day; the number of ORS packets distributed at a clinic indicates how many mothers heard the ORT message.

Behavioral products observation is particularly useful when direct observation of a target behavior cannot be made or is too time-consuming or when direct observation might make a person respond differently (Barlow, Hayes, & Nelson, 1984). For example, one of the principal questions in ORS utilization is the quantity of solution actually administered to the child in the home. Studies conducted in Mexico and Lesotho (Touchette, Elder, & Nagiel, 1990) demonstrated that the amount of ORS used in the home could be directly measured and used to corroborate mothers' verbal reports. Mothers were provided a liter of premixed ORS solution in the clinic and were requested to administer all of the solution to their children within the next twenty-four hours. Observers then visited the mothers in their homes the next day and measured the amount of ORS solution left in the bottle. (See Exhibit 3.6.)

Exhibit 3.6. Home ORS Administration Observation.

Home #	*Child's Age*	*Weight*	*Amount of ORS Remaining*
1	3 mos.	4.8 kg	700 ml
2	33 mos.	13.4 kg	450 ml
3	6 mos.	6.7 kg	600 ml
4	20 mos.	12.6 kg	200 ml

Generally, in behavioral products observation, the observer simply records the site and the number or amount of products observed. Growth monitoring is another example of behavior products observation. In Exhibit 3.7, the health worker is observing the outcome of weaning and breast-feeding behaviors by measuring the weight of the child. In growth-monitoring programs, children are weighed every month, and clinic and/or village health workers record the child's weight on a "growth chart," which is used to help parents understand whether their child is growing appropriately.

Home or Clinic Trial Observation. Observation conducted at homes or in clinics is designed to test target behaviors with a small number of the target audience before the behaviors are promoted on a massive scale. Just as communicators pretest broadcast and print material with the target audience, they should test target behaviors as well. Once again, the focus is on actually observing target behaviors and noting how the target audience adapts them to "real life." In home or clinic trials, the researcher teaches a person how to perform a behavior and asks him or her to continue performing it for several days. The researcher then revisits the person, to observe the behavior being performed and to discuss how the person has adapted it (see Touchette, Elder, & Nagiel, 1990). This technique enables communicators to develop a detailed list of steps for performing the behavior and to identify and understand the antecedents that trigger the behaviors and the consequences that result when these behaviors are performed in "real life."

This technique is particularly useful in trials of new practices or behaviors. For instance, in introducing a new weaning food,

Exhibit 3.7. A Growth-Monitoring Chart.

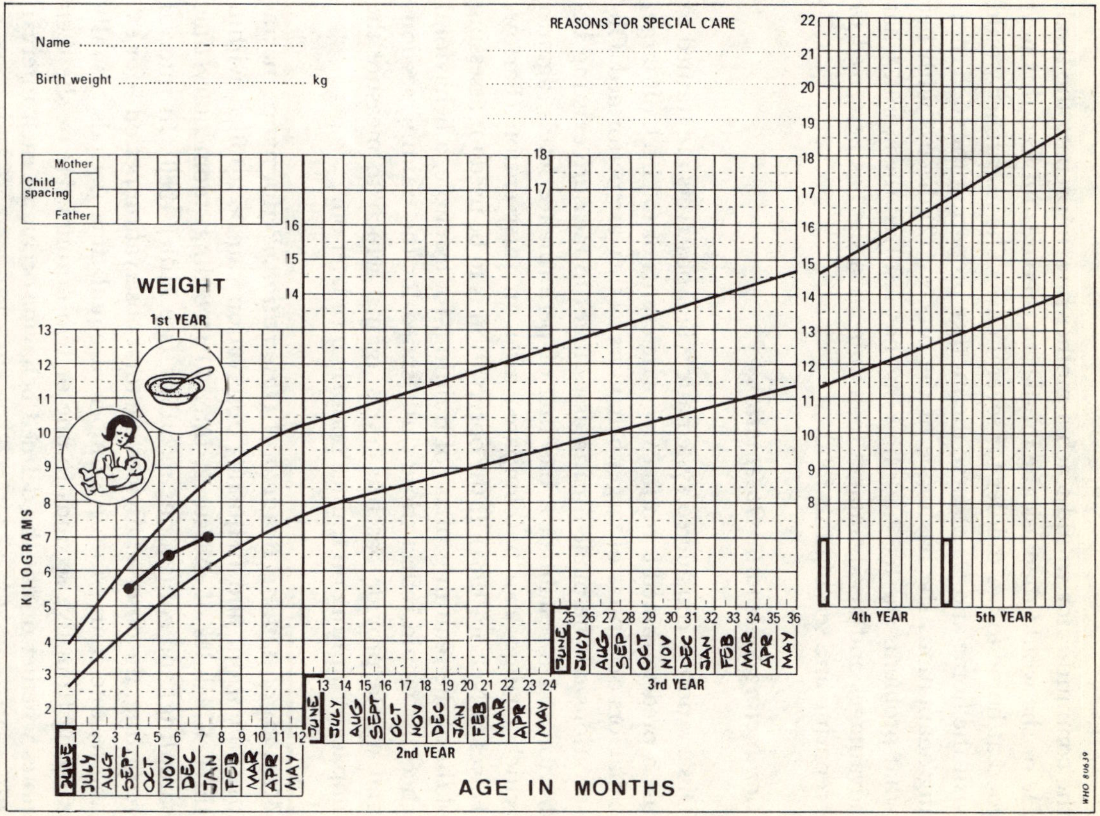

Source: Reproduced, by permission, from *The growth chart: A tool for use in infant and child health care.* Geneva, World Health Organization, 1986, Fig. 2, p. 12, and Fig. 12, p. 21.

the communicator would teach a mother how to prepare the food. He or she would then ask the mother to prepare and feed this new food at home to her toddler for several days. The researcher would visit the home and (1) observe the mother preparing the food, noting adaptations she has made in the process; (2) discuss with her what problems she has had, how she has resolved them, and what advantages and disadvantages (consequences) she has perceived in preparing and serving this food.

Conducting Systematic Observations

Observation is considered systematic when observers are trained to use a predetermined form to categorize events or to check off target behaviors or aspects of target behaviors as they are performed. Observations can be made during assessment to measure existing behavior and to establish a baseline of performance levels, against which changes can be compared after an intervention (Barlow, Hayes, & Nelson, 1984). If the observation is to be used for assessing skills at the planning phase of training, for example, a behavioral checklist would reflect those skills slated for the training sessions and would provide baseline levels against which to measure the impact of training on trainee performance later on.

Methods of Timing Behavioral Observation. Performance, narrative, duration, and frequency observation can be applied within three schedules of measures: interval recording, momentary time sampling, and continuous recording (see Miller 1980). In interval recording, the observer divides the total observation period—for example, one hour—into a number of equal time periods, usually ranging from five seconds to one or two minutes. He or she then notes whether or not the defined behavior occurs in each interval. Interval length should be such that the behavior typically occurs only once in each interval. In momentary time sampling, the observer takes brief "snapshot" observations throughout the designated time period. These snapshots can be evenly spaced or random. For example, to find out how many women are standing in line outside of clinics, an observer can conduct momentary time sampling on an hourly basis; such a sampling can provide a reliable daily average. In continuous recording, the observer applies the technique during a continuous period of observation.

In choosing the best timing for observation, communicators should take into consideration who is going to perform the observation, what will be recorded, and when and how often it is to be recorded. As a rule of thumb, if the behavior occurs fairly infrequently (less than several times a day), each instance should be recorded during continuous observation; if the behavior occurs very frequently (many times a day), momentary or interval recording can be used; if the quality of practice hinges on how long it lasts, its duration should be recorded (Rasmuson, Seidel, Smith, & Booth, 1988).

Developing a Behavioral Observation Form. Observation forms are designed to systematize the observation of behavior. In narrative recording, a sheet divided into thirds—with headings of "Antecedent," "Behavior," "Consequence"—will be enough to organize a trained observer's responses. On the other hand, as demonstrated above, performance, duration, frequency, and behavioral products observation forms are based on a predetermined list of ideal behaviors or behavioral steps and/or physical products to be observed.

In making up a checklist, researchers should express all items as observable events. For example, although "Encourages mothers to participate" is an important aspect of an effective health talk, "encourage" is not just one behavior and is not directly observable. The concept, therefore, must be broken down to describe what a health worker actually does "to encourage"—for example, "Asks individual mothers a question," "Uses a mother in a demonstration," "Praises mother," "Smiles and nods when a mother responds."

Phrasing items on the checklist in terms of observable behavior helps to reduce the amount of interpretation observers need to rate performance. Observers might interpret "Encourages mothers" in very different ways, because they might be looking for different signs of that encouragement. Breaking down "encouragement" into specific actions, such as "Smiles and nods when a mother responds" and "Praises mothers," helps ensure that each observer will look specifically at those actions when rating the general area of encouragement. However, the checklist should not be too long or it will be unwieldy to apply. Only a few "encourage" or other similar general behaviors should be selected for observers to check.

Adding follow-up questions helps to flesh out the strictly quantitative aspect of the checklist. Additional open-ended questions allow the observer to comment on conditions that might affect the person's regular performance or to give information about frequently occurring related behaviors not on the checklist.

Selecting Observers. Observational researchers must be carefully selected, since the validity of the data gathered relies primarily on the quality of the observation. Sometimes people directly involved in the program would be best at conducting the observations. For example, nurses and doctors can observe clinic practices. Not only will they learn from observing, but the process will make them feel more involved in the program and more likely to use the data to undertake changes in clinic procedures. If the behavior is a private one, the person performing it might be able to record his or her own behavior. For example, a mother—if she is known to be reliable—may be able to keep track of how many times she breast-feeds in twenty-four hours. Generally, however, communicators will wish to use neutral, outside observers who are not biased and can be selected for specific qualities that make for good researchers: interest, patience, neutrality, attention to detail, reliability, resourcefulness, and practical experience. Teachers, social workers, or college and university students with these qualities might make competent outside observers.

Training Observers. Regardless of which technique is selected, observers must be carefully trained in the use of the observation instrument. They must become comfortable with the format through repeated practice; and, most important, they must agree on what sets of actions constitute the behaviors targeted for observation and record behaviors in the same way. During training, observers review the checklist and agree on what behaviors constitute each item. They then observe several role plays and compare their results as a group (agreements and disagreements) item by item.

The issue of language is also important to cover in training observers. If the instrument is written and the training session conducted in the consultant's or the country's official language (for instance, in French, English, or Spanish) but the people in the setting where the behaviors are observed will be using another language, training should be conducted in both; observer agreements also should be measured in both instances. In Zaire, where health workers giving health talks in Swahili were to be observed, observer training occurred in both French and Swahili. Initially, health talks were role-played in French, so that the communicators, some of whom did not speak Swahili, and observers could discuss how well instrument items reflected the actual behaviors they were to observe. Later, when the observers were agreeing 90 percent on their ratings and the communicators felt that the instrument needed no further revision, they role-played the health talks in Swahili, to simulate more closely the actual sessions where the instruments would be applied. Initially, observers' accuracy fell off until they became accustomed to hearing health content areas correctly presented in Swahili.

Monitoring Observers. Once the research is under way, observers must be monitored periodically to ensure that the data they are collecting are reliable and accurate. The supervisor should conduct spot interobserver reliability checks by asking two researchers to observe the same activity and comparing the scoring on their instruments. Their data are considered reliable if they agree on 80 percent or more of the items. Reliability checks should be carried out on 25–30 percent of the total number of observations (see Miller, 1980).

Graphing Results. Results from observational research can be easily graphed in order to provide a simple picture of what is happening to the behavior over time. Graphing observational data during the assessment phase will create a baseline for a program; these data can then be compared with data collected once an intervention is under way. The techniques and applications of graphing are further discussed in Chapter Six.

Summary

Assessment is the first stage of the communication process. During this stage, communicators gather information in order to plan communication strategies based on the needs, cultural context, and practices of the target audience. They gather this information by beginning a dialogue with the community through research with representatives of the target audience. In this way, communicators shift the focus from the technical issues of the medical problem to what people need to *do* to respond to the health problem.

To plan a behaviorally focused communication program, communicators should define the "ideal" (medically correct) behavior and compare it to existing behaviors of the target audience. A series of questions about existing behavior—such as which behaviors compete with the ideal behavior, which ones are approximations, and whether the absence of ideal behavior is due to a skills deficit or a performance deficit—will help communicators design strategies to strengthen, replace, teach, or maintain those behaviors.

Critical to the planning process are questions about what consequences exist for both ideal and competing behaviors. To help answer these questions, communicators can add questions to research instruments to identify consequences as well as observe the behaviors directly. They can then specifically design programs with consequences that support performance of desired behaviors.

4

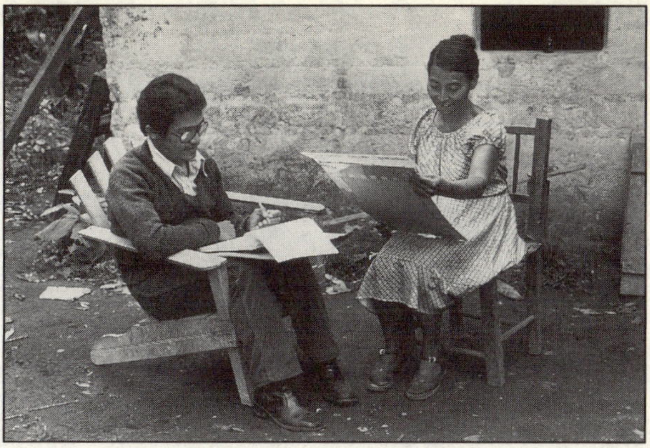

Planning for Behavior Change

During planning, communicators use primary and secondary research results to segment target audiences; select behaviors; plan strategies; develop messages; and design management, distribution, monitoring, and evaluation systems (Debus, 1988). This chapter focuses on how the communicator analyzes the relationships between the environment and the desired behaviors and takes those relationships into consideration when selecting target behaviors, planning communication strategies, and selecting communication channels. Specifically, this chapter describes the behavioral approach to selecting target behaviors that are most amenable to change and have the greatest potential impact on the health problem and organizing them in order of priority; developing communication strategies that remedy skills and performance deficits by teaching and supporting skills development and creating an environment of support for maintaining learned behaviors; selecting integrated interpersonal, print, and mass media channels to function as consequences as well as antecedents to target behaviors.

Selecting Target Behaviors

The selection of target behaviors is one of the most difficult decisions made during planning. Traditionally, communicators, in an effort to provide comprehensive information on the health problem, have included too many behaviors and messages in their programs; the result is very little impact on behavior change. Communication programs that have achieved behavior change have focused on a limited number of feasible behaviors. For example, in a successful immunization program in the Philippines, communication messages focused exclusively on motivating parents to obtain the measles vaccination by the time their child was nine months old. Other immunizations were not mentioned in the communication messages to the target audience. Nonetheless, health workers were taught to use this opportunity to bring all children up to date on all immunizations when they arrived for the measles vaccination. During the six-month nationwide urban measles intervention, conducted in 1990, measles immunization coverage of nine- to twenty-three-month-old children increased significantly, from 54 percent to 68 percent. Complete immunization coverage for children between nine and eleven months old also increased significantly, from 33 percent to more than 56 percent (Seidel, 1992). To achieve behavior change, therefore, communicators must eliminate the majority of the "ideal behaviors" and select a core of feasible target behaviors as the focus of their communication program.

There are several reasons why communicators should establish a short list of behaviors to promote. First, behaviors related to desired health practices are frequently too numerous and complex to introduce, change, and maintain all at one time. Second, some behaviors are more easily changed than others; some behaviors are simply not feasible for the target audience to perform, and others are incompatible with social and cultural norms. Third, some behaviors have more potential impact on the health problem. Communication programs sometimes have promoted behaviors that have no clearly demonstrated relationship to the specific health problem. For example, although boiling water is an important behavior to prevent infant diarrhea, it is not a necessary step to treat dehydration. Boiled water has little impact on the efficacy of rehydration, and the high cost in time and resources required to boil and cool the water may actually deter the mother from using ORS.

Steps in Selecting Behaviors

The following steps will help communicators select a few key behaviors to be targets for a communication program.

Step 1: Review Assessment Research. The planning process begins with a review of the data concerning a target audience's current beliefs, knowledge, and practices related to the health problem. This review will help planners understand existing behaviors and the consequences that maintain them, and to decide which behaviors are really feasible for the target audience to adopt.

Step 2: Review the List of "Ideal" Behaviors. Ideal behaviors are the medically prescribed behavioral steps that the target audience should perform in order to prevent or treat the health problem. As described in Chapter Three, in the assessment stage, an interdisciplinary team initiates the definition of the ideal behavior. During the planning stage, the team reviews its list of "ideal" behaviors and adds steps that assessment research has identified as appropriate and necessary for the correct performance and maintenance of the health practice. For example, in a vitamin A program, researchers may have found that mothers were already preparing a food rich in this vitamin and that this particular food did not appear on the team's original list.

Step 3: Select Target Behaviors. Target behaviors are the minimum number of behavioral steps essential for the health practice to be effective. All unnecessary and unfeasible behaviors and behavioral steps must first be excluded from the ideal behavior list, so that the list is reduced to a manageable core, which will be the focus of the communication program.

As illustrated in Figure 4.1, the selection of target behaviors is a process of elimination. The planning team includes existing approximations and excludes behaviors that have no demonstrated impact on the specific health problem and are not feasible for the target audience to adopt. The final target behaviors of the commu-

Figure 4.1. Selecting Target Behaviors: Playing the Elimination Game.

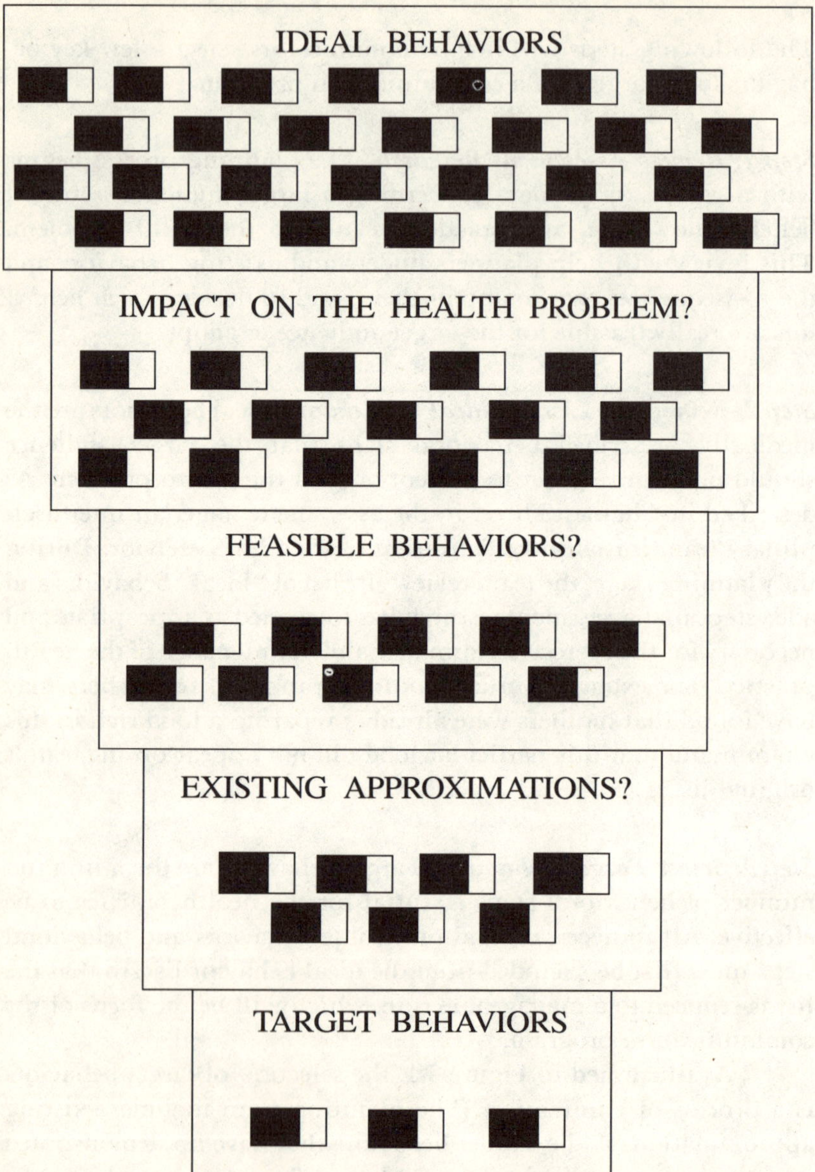

nication program will be a highly selective subset of the medically prescribed ideal behaviors defined during assessment.

During the process of elimination, the planning team considers the health impact and feasibility of each ideal behavior, as well as the approximations to that behavior that are already being performed by the target audience. The following questions can assist the team in honing the long list of ideal behaviors down to the core set of target behaviors:

1. *Does the ideal behavior have a demonstrated impact on this specific health problem?* If it does not, it should not be selected as a target behavior.
2. *Is the ideal behavior feasible for the audience to perform?* An in-depth understanding of the target audience is essential if one is to understand the environmental constraints that will affect adoption.
   - Does the ideal behavior produce negative consequences for the person performing it?
   - Is the ideal behavior incompatible with the person's current behavior or with sociocultural norms or acceptable practices?
   - Does the ideal behavior require an unrealistic rate of frequency?
   - Does the ideal behavior require an unrealistic duration?
   - Does the ideal behavior have too high a cost in time, energy, social status, money, or materials?
   - Is the ideal behavior too complex and not easily divided into a small number of elements or steps?
3. *Are any existing behaviors approximations to the ideal behavior?* Can these behaviors be shaped into an effective health practice through training and skill development? Communication programs are more likely to achieve behavior change if they build on what people are already doing correctly. If existing behaviors are similar to any of the remaining ideal behaviors, they should be included in the list of target behaviors.

The team will need to be very discerning and make some hard decisions by weighing the pros and cons of each behavior. A behavior might be necessary to have an impact on health, but it may be impossible for people to carry out. For example, in an acute respiratory infection program, one ideal behavior proposed during assessment was that parents use vaporizers to produce steam for children to inhale. However, formative research indicated that most homes, particularly those of children most at risk, did not have electricity. In other cases, a behavior might be feasible, but it would not really have an impact on the health problem. The ARI planning team had also considered the alternative of having mothers boil water on the stove to produce steam. The formative research indicated, however, that, although mothers did not have problems performing this behavior, it would not have any impact because windows were left open to provide light, and the steam would escape before it could have any effect. As a result, vaporization was eliminated from the list of target behaviors.

This process of elimination is not necessarily either-or but, rather, a balancing of all the factors that might determine whether or not a behavior will be adopted. Sometimes the behaviors are not feasible for the target audience to perform in their ideal form, but they are absolutely necessary to have an impact on the health problem. In this case, the team enters into a process of negotiation with a medical or nutritional specialist, to try to find some intermediate point between the ideal and existing behaviors that could still have some health impact. For example, if a behavior requires too high a frequency, duration, or cost in its ideal form, the team will need to negotiate with a medical specialist a way to reduce that frequency, duration, or cost. In the Guatemala hand-washing program, the planning team concluded that mothers should wash their hands twenty-six times a day, and each hand washing required an average of 600 cc of water and approximately two minutes of time. In this case, the ideal behavior obviously had too high a cost for the target audience. The team negotiated with the epidemiologist in order to determine the times when hand washing could have the most impact on diarrhea morbidity. As a result, the list of target behaviors was reduced to two: hand washing before preparing meals and before administering foods to children under three years old.

At this point the team may need to return to the target audience, to test its reaction to any new behaviors on the list. Asking for opinions and reactions in focus-group discussions or, better still, observing actual trials of the behaviors will help planners come up with a final list of desired behaviors. In Guatemala, the planning team first listed (selected) ten health practices for promotion related to feeding during diarrhea. They used this process of elimination to reduce the list from ten to four. They then tested each of the four behaviors in five home trials. The data from the home trials helped them finally select one behavior as the focus of the communication program.

If the list of target behaviors is still too numerous to be manageable, the team will need to determine which behaviors should be focused on initially and which can be introduced later in the program. This shortened list of essential target behaviors allows the team to select communication strategies, communication channels, training objectives, monitoring tools, and program evaluation criteria to focus more explicitly and effectively on behavior change early in the program. Later, communicators can introduce target behaviors more critical to maintaining the health practice.

Tools for Selecting Behaviors

The Behavior Analysis Scale (adapted from Green, Kreuter, Deeds, Partridge, 1980) is particularly useful when a health practice is the target for communication for the first time. (For a sample of the scale and a more detailed explanation of how to use it, see Resource E.) The scale includes nine criteria of behavior against which a potential target behavior can be rated: impact on the health problem, positive consequences, compatibility, frequency, duration, cost, approximations, complexity, and observability. The interdisciplinary team rates each behavioral step from 0 to 5 for each criterion. The resulting "score" helps planners see which of many behaviors are most amenable to change and which have the most potential for impact on the health problem. The Behavior Analysis Scale is not a rigorous scientific methodology. Indeed, the interdisciplinary team may find that, even with research results, they still have to score items without data or with available information that is contradictory. The ratings frequently reflect a compromise among the various disciplines represented on the team. Nevertheless, the scale offers a coherent guide to select target behaviors, permitting all of the principal concerns from a variety of disciplines to be discussed systematically.

Target Behavior Selection Worksheets (Mata, 1992) were successfully used in a Peruvian communication program. (For samples of these worksheets and a more complete description of how to use them, see Resource F.) An interdisciplinary team completes the Technically Ideal Behavioral Profile and the Existing Behavioral Profile worksheets; during planning, an interdisciplinary team compares the two and completes the Target Behavioral Profile worksheet. Each worksheet is organized into five columns: the behavior, the reason for performing it, the benefit (or consequence) from performing it, its cost, and the vocabulary used to describe the behavior.

To select the target behaviors, the interdisciplinary team first decides which behaviors on the Ideal Behavioral Profile worksheet do not have any demonstrated impact on the selected health problem; these items are not considered as behaviors. Team members then compare ideal and existing behaviors and analyze where they are the same, where approximations exist, and where the two are completely different. The behaviors on the two worksheets that are the same and are approximations are selected as target behaviors. In situations where ideal behaviors are radically different from what the target audience is currently doing, but are necessary for impact on the health problem, the team enters into negotiation with a medical specialist to determine a more feasible intermediate target behavior. Again, this is not a scientifically rigorous methodology, but it assists the planning team in organizing discussions.

Selecting Communication Strategies

Communicators must consider many factors—medical, political, financial, logistical, and technical—when deciding on the "best" communication strategy. Behavioral factors also should play a part in influencing strategy selection. This section describes how communicators analyze the relationships between the environment and desired behaviors and take those relationships into consideration when selecting communication strategies.

Skills and Performance Deficits

In selecting communication strategies, communicators should consider whether the absence or incorrect performance of a target behavior is due to a lack of skills (skills deficit) or the absence of conditions favorable for performing it (performance deficit) (Bandura, 1977; Miller, 1980; Sulzer-Azaroff & Mayer, 1977). When the person has a skills deficit, communicators will select strategies to introduce and teach these skills. If the audience is already performing approximations to the target behaviors, the communication strategy will reward those approximations and teach the skills necessary to shape them into target behaviors.

In other instances, people have significant knowledge and skills, but they are still not performing the behavior correctly or at all. One reason may be that performing the behavior does not produce any immediately perceivable consequences or may actually produce unpleasant consequences. In this case, the communication strategy will focus less on teaching skills and shaping behavior and more on developing an environment of support for continued performance of the target behavior. For example, community-based primary health care volunteers, who are vital channels of interpersonal communication to mothers and other caretakers, generally receive some training and initially have an acceptable level of skills to provide basic health services and information at the community level (Werner & Bower, 1976). Despite a good beginning, however, attrition rates for these volunteers are high throughout the developing world, and their potential impact as conduits of health information, skills, and reinforcement to their communities is greatly diminished (Elder, et al., 1992). Frequently, program planners conclude that community health workers need more training to "keep them motivated." The problem here, however, is more a performance than a skills deficit. An analysis of the situation from a behavioral perspective would lead to a strategy focusing less on retraining and skill building and more on increasing pleasant consequences and decreasing unpleasant consequences for the volunteers' work. Research would be used to determine which consequences would be most likely to increase desired behaviors and which unpleasant consequences might be decreased. This information would be used in the design of a support system to help these workers continue to be effective and active volunteers.

Performance deficits are also a common problem when mothers fail to perform target behaviors correctly. Once again, a communication strategy would focus less on skill building and more on creating an environment of support (Kyenkya-Isabirye & Magalheas, 1990). Research could be used to identify what unpleasant consequences might be deterring this practice or whether it produces few, if any, pleasant consequences. For example, many mothers are convinced that breast feeding is best for their infants and are taught how to breast-feed at the hospital. Breast feeding can be extremely painful, however, particularly in the first several weeks. First-time mothers, in spite of their good intentions and skills, may feel overwhelmed and frustrated by this pain. The communication strategy in this case could focus on increasing social support during the first month of breast feeding. Communication could be used to teach fathers and other women how to support the first-time mother during this initial month.

Decisions for Strategy Selection

The flow chart shown as Figure 4.2 is a decision tree that can assist communicators in selecting communication strategies. It is divided into two general areas: skills deficit (on the left-hand side) and performance deficit (on the right). To use the flow chart, communicators first consider whether people know about the target behavior. If they do not, communicators generally will select antecedent strategies to introduce a behavior, provide information, and create awareness of and demand for new health technologies and behaviors. For example, in the early days of diarrheal disease control, most ORT communication strategies first focused on introducing the concept of dehydration and the need for ORS to prevent deaths from dehydration.

If people are aware of the behavior, communicators would then consider whether "people are able to perform the behavior if they are asked." If not, they have a skills deficit, and communicators would select strategies to train and teach skills and to shape approximations.

Figure 4.2. Selecting Communication Strategies: Decision Tree.

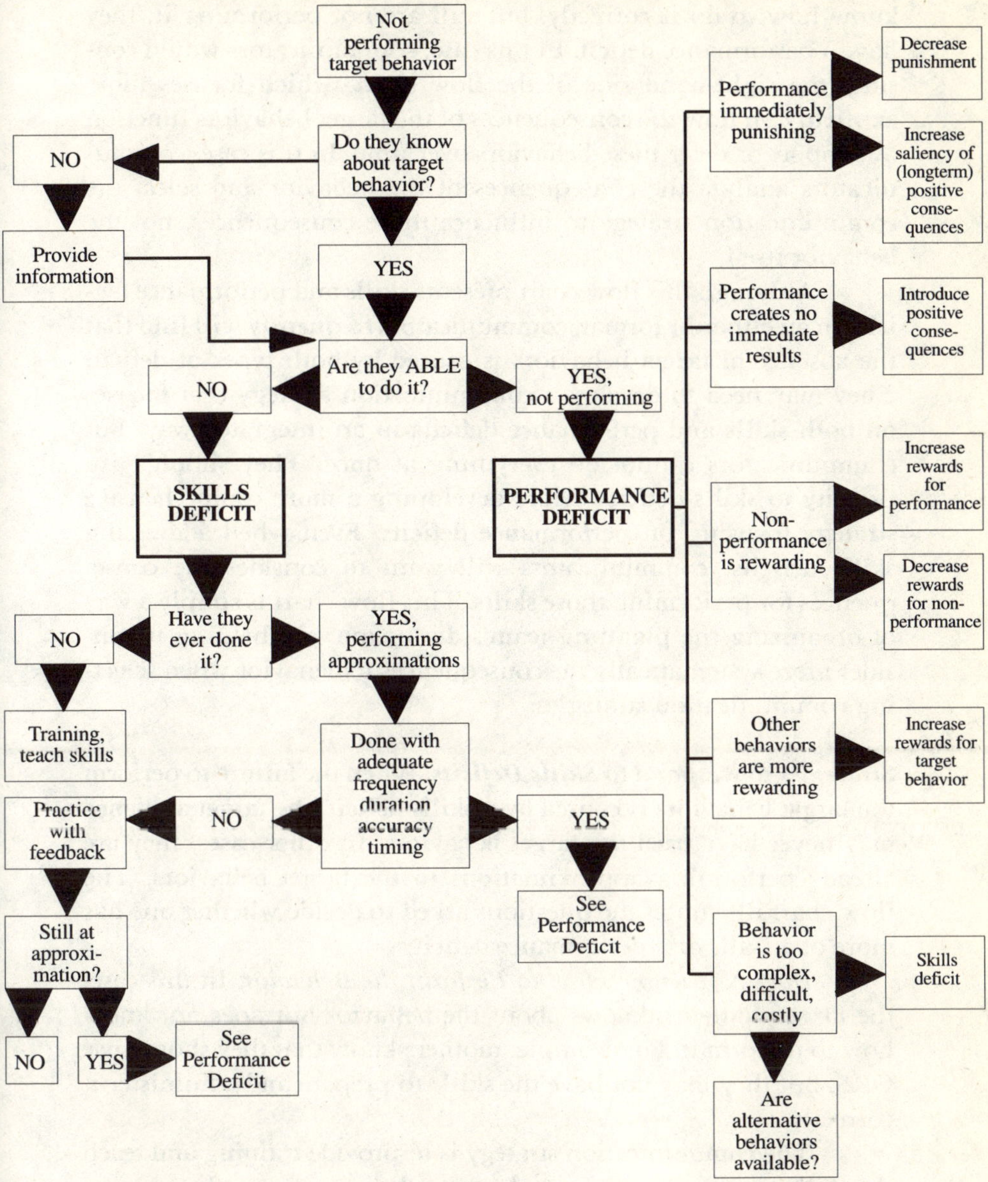

Source: Adapted from the Flow Diagram in *Analyzing Performance Problems,* Mager & Pipe, Second Edition, 1984, p. 3. Copyright © 1984 by Lake Publishing Company, Belmont, CA 94002.

If, on the other hand, people know about the behavior and know how to do it correctly, but still are not performing it, they have a performance deficit. In this case, communicators would consider the right-hand side of the flow chart, which focuses more explicitly on how the consequences of the target behaviors function to support or deter these behaviors over time. In this case, communicators analyze the consequences of the behavior and select the communication strategy to influence those consequences, not the behavior itself.

Although this flow chart presents skills and performance deficits in an either-or format, communicators frequently will find that the absence of target behaviors is caused by both types of deficit. They may need to develop a communication strategy that focuses on both skills and performance deficits in an integrated way. But communicators cannot do everything at once. They should give priority to skills deficits before developing a more comprehensive strategy focusing on performance deficits. Even when addressing skills deficits, communicators will want to consider the consequences for performing those skills. This flow chart is simply a way of organizing the planning team's discussion and helping it consider more systematically the consequences to behavior when selecting communication strategies.

Strategies to Respond to Skills Deficits. When the failure to perform the target behaviors is caused by a skills deficit, the target audience may never have tried the target behaviors. In other cases, they are already performing approximations to the target behaviors. The flow chart illustrates the questions asked to decide whether one has more of a skills or a performance deficit.

Does Not Know How to Perform the Behavior. In this case, the target audience knows about the behavior but does not know how to perform it. For example, mothers know that they should use ORS, but they may not have the skills to prepare and administer it correctly.

The communication strategy is to provide training and teach the skills necessary to perform the target behavior correctly.

Performs Approximations to the Behavior. In this case, the target audience is performing approximations to the target behavior, but not in sufficient frequency, duration, the correct form, or at the right time.

The communication strategy is to reward approximations and teach correct frequency, duration, accuracy, and timing (Mager & Pipe, 1984).

Strategies to Respond to Performance Deficits. In other instances, as mentioned, most people in the target audience can demonstrate how to perform the target behavior correctly, but still are not performing it in their daily lives. For example, many people can demonstrate correct hand washing, but still do not wash their hands during the day because consequences deter or do not support that behavior. The communicator then looks to the right side of the flow chart and begins to consider why this performance deficit exists.

When considering strategies to address performance deficits, the communicator needs to recognize that a behavior leads to more than one consequence. A behavior can actually produce a wide range of consequences—from positive to negative, from immediate to delayed, and from concrete to abstract. Communicators might want to start their strategy selection by listing all the consequences that, according to formative research, occur when a person performs or does not perform the behavior. This list can help communicators organize their discussion and select the most effective way to use those consequences to support target behaviors. Consequences that are culturally relevant, individually salient, and immediate will be the most powerful. Delayed or abstract consequences are much less so. For example, communicators have frequently promoted certain weaning foods or preventive practices such as immunizations by saying "They will keep your child healthy." A "healthy child" is, of course, a positive outcome that all parents desire, but it is a vague and delayed notion and not clearly linked to any one behavior. The most effective communication strategy emphasizes positive consequences and also selects consequences that people recognize as being closely linked to their behavior.

Some negative consequences, such as the pain caused by breast feeding or side effects of medication, cannot be eliminated by a communication program; nevertheless, a creative communicator can develop ways to lessen the impact of this punishment by focusing on other consequences. The following sections provide examples of communication strategies that respond to performance deficits.

When Performance Is Immediately Punishing. In this case, a person actually receives perceptible punishment for performing a behavior. The punishment may come from individuals in his or her social network. For example, a husband may be unhappy if dinner is not ready because his wife took their child for immunizations, or grandmothers may disapprove of a mother for feeding a child differently during weaning. In other instances, punishment may come from the health system: doctors may scold mothers for waiting too long to bring their children to the clinic when they are ill. Finally, punishment can come from performing the behavior itself: ORS, if administered too rapidly, can cause vomiting.

The communication strategy is to decrease unpleasant consequences and/or increase the saliency of positive ones. To decrease an unpleasant consequence, communicators must first determine where the punishment is coming from and then develop strategies to change or lower the impact of this punishment. For example, if the punishment is coming from a husband, he could be encouraged to take more of a role in the children's immunization, so that he will be less critical of the mother's practice. If the punishment is coming from the behavior itself, communicators may want to develop a strategy to incorporate or strengthen another salient source to provide positive consequences. For example, breast feeding can be perceived to have an immediately punishing consequence. It can be extremely painful, especially during the first weeks. It also requires a good deal of a mother's time and patience, and some mothers complain that it restricts their movements and keeps them from other responsibilities. To decrease the power of these unpleasant consequences, a breast-feeding communication strategy could prepare a mother for the immediate consequences and urge women in the family and neighborhood to provide extra encouragement during this period. Eventually, the pain lessens, and the naturally occurring benefits of breast feeding take effect and support the behavior. Communicators also could encourage older children or other family members to support the mother by running errands or caring for the other children while she is breast-feeding.

When Performance Creates No Immediate Results. Because of their preventive nature, many target behaviors aimed at child survival have no immediate, salient consequences that the person performing the behavior can easily perceive. For example, a mother may not be able to see that, because of her new feeding practices, her child is maintaining his weight during a diarrhea episode.

The communication strategy is to introduce new positive consequences for behavior. The communication strategy might introduce planned consequences in order to support the behavior until naturally occurring consequences are perceived. Material consequences could be introduced; for instance, diplomas or prizes could be given to mothers whose children maintain their weight in spite of diarrheal episodes. Or communicators might incorporate social consequences into the strategy by changing other people's behavior to create an environment of support for the mother; they might, for example, ask a husband to congratulate his wife or a mother-in-law to praise her daughter-in-law for feeding practices during diarrheal episodes. It is also possible to teach the individual to recognize new, more immediate consequences for his or her own behavior (Miller, 1980; Baer, Wolf, & Risley, 1968; Sulzer-Azaroff & Mayer, 1977). For example, a mother might be asked to use a colorful calendar to record how many times her sick child eats during a day.

If a communication program introduces planned consequences, communicators will also need to develop antecedent strategies to increase the saliency of the new consequence. In the examples above, mothers would be informed that prizes and diplomas are available; mothers-in-law would be taught how and when to congratulate their daughters-in-law; and mothers would be taught how to use the calendar.

As discussed, the choice of the most culturally appropriate, personally salient, and immediate consequence to introduce should be guided by research with the specific target audience. What communicators may deem as the "best" consequence may not be the one perceived as "best" by the target audience. For example, in the villages of Central Java, Indonesia, dropout rates of volunteer primary health care workers were extremely high. Communicators used focus-group research to find out what consequences would be most likely to support these volunteers in continuing their work.

The communicators had thought that material rewards, such as T-shirts and diplomas, would be selected, and these options were presented and discussed during the focus groups. The health care workers said, however, that public acknowledgment from village leaders would be the most rewarding consequence for their work—a consequence that the communicators had not even considered before conducting the research (Reis, Elder, Satoto, Kodyat, & Palmer, 1990).

Communicators also must consider how the planned consequences they introduce will be phased out over time and what naturally occurring consequences will take their place. For the long-term performance of behavior, communicators cannot rely on planned consequences. The maintenance of behavior change is discussed further in Chapter Seven.

When Nonperformance Is More Rewarding Than Performance. In many instances, the household responsibilities of children's caretakers compete with their performance of many health practices. For example, when she does *not* take a child to be immunized, the mother has more time to work in the family garden and does not have to arrange care for the other children left at home. In this way, she is actually rewarded for *not* immunizing her child.

The communication strategy is to increase rewards for the target behaviors. Caretakers often have not experienced any positive consequences from performing a target behavior such as obtaining immunizations several times over the first year of a child's life. In order to make the immunization process more attractive to and feasible for a mother, the communication strategy would combine actual changes in clinic practices with communication messages to promote clinic services. Clinics would try to make visits more positive through better service (faster, more polite), better care, and motivational schemes (diplomas, lotteries). After experiencing more positive consequences from the behavior, the mother is more likely *to do* rather than *not to do*.

When Other Behaviors Are More Rewarding. In child survival programs, mothers frequently perform behaviors deemed counterproductive for the health of their children. For example, mothers bottle-feed rather than breast-feed.

The communication strategy is to increase rewards for the

target behavior or increase punishment for undesired behaviors. Communicators generally prefer to develop strategies that increase rewards for the target behaviors. Rather than openly attacking mothers' existing practices, the communication strategy promotes a new practice that directly competes with it. In Honduras, the Ministry of Health's breast-feeding program promoted breast milk as the most healthy, complete, and sanitary food for infants rather than decrying formula (Booth, 1985). Communicators could also consider a strategy to increase negative consequences or punishment for a competing or nondesired behavior, but this strategy generally has not been used in public health programs in developing countries.

When Behavior Is Too Complex, Difficult, or Costly. In this case, (1) the interdisciplinary team has selected target behaviors that are not feasible because of high cost, complexity, or difficulty; or (2) the target audience still does not know *how* to perform the behavior correctly (a skills deficit). If (1), the team must return to the step of selecting target behaviors. If (2), communicators must return to the left-hand side of the flow chart to select their communication strategy.

Case Study: Selecting Target Behaviors and Communication Strategies in a Guatemalan Water and Sanitation Program

As described in the case study in Chapter Three, the Nutrition Institute for Central America and Panama (INCAP) received funding from the World Health Organization to implement a communication program designed to lower diarrheal morbidity through increased use of a newly installed community water system. An interdisciplinary team made up of an epidemiologist, a physician, two health communicators, a regional health trainer, and an anthropologist met to define the ideal behavior and areas of formative research to be conducted during assessment. Through this analysis, the team defined "correct hand washing" as the health practice to be promoted by the program, defined the behavioral steps necessary to perform "ideal" hand washing, and concluded that hand washing was both complex and costly to mothers, the primary audience of the program. The team members realized that they needed to lower this cost and decided to use home trials to test the Tippy-Tap, a simple hand-washing device originally developed in Africa. This device reduces the amount of water needed for hand washing and at the same time is an attractive new technology that could motivate this health practice. However, fifty-four behavioral steps were identified for the fabrication, installation, and maintenance of the Tippy-Tap. The team therefore decided to use in-depth interviews and focus-group discussions to understand how other family members could be incorporated into the communication strategy to perform some of the steps needed to make, install, and maintain this device.

After conducting formative research during the assessment stage, the interdisciplinary team met again to use the results to select target behaviors and develop communication strategies necessary to increase correct hand washing. Since this was the first time communication had been applied to a water and sanitation program by the institute, the team used the Behavior Analysis Scale to select target behaviors. The discussions were lively as each discipline presented its rationale for the scores. The epidemiologist assessed the potential impact of each step on the health problem—diarrheal morbidity. At the same time, the anthropologist and the social science researcher looked closely at behavioral approximations, compatibility, and the cost of the behavioral steps to mothers, compared with what they were already doing. Application of the Behavior Analysis Scale helped the team reduce the target hand-washing behaviors from fifty-four to twenty-two.

The team members then moved to developing the communication strategy. They decided that the health practice was not being performed because of a performance deficit. That is, mothers found it too costly to perform all the behavioral steps necessary for "correct hand washing." The communication strategy, therefore, focused on decreasing the unpleasant consequences of hand washing by systematically incorporating fathers and older siblings in installing and maintaining the Tippy-Tap and helping mothers wash younger children's hands. The strategy also focused on increasing pleasant consequences by asking family members to congratulate or thank each other for washing infants' hands.

Selecting Communication Channels

After communicators have selected target behaviors and defined communication strategies, they can select the messages and channels to be used to communicate to the target audience. In child survival programs, the various communication channels are usually referred to as interpersonal, broadcast, and print channels. Each channel has its own strengths and weaknesses, depending on the role it will take in the communication program. But communication strategies that combine multiple channels have the most impact on changing health behavior (United States Department of Health and Human Services, 1989). The question is no longer which channel is the best but, rather, how to use a combination of channels to teach and support target behaviors.

- *Interpersonal channels*—such as face-to-face communication, community distribution, home visits, training, group discussions, and counseling—are generally best for giving credibility to messages, providing information, and teaching complex skills that need two-way communication between the individual and a credible source of information. Interpersonal communication facilitates the discussion of information or messages that the target audience regards as "sensitive" or "personal." It is also important for providing positive feedback and immediate reinforcement to the people performing the target behaviors.
- *Broadcast channels* generally provide broad coverage for communication messages, reaching a large number of the target audience quickly and frequently. In developing countries, radio has been a powerful channel to reach large numbers of people with communication messages, and to model target behaviors and their consequences. In some countries, such as Egypt and the Philippines, television has also played an important role.
- *Print channels*—such as pamphlets, flyers, and posters—are

generally considered best for providing a timely reminder of key communication messages. Pamphlets and other graphic materials distributed at the individual or home level can provide complex information in a digestible form, so that the target audience can use that information when it most needs it. Audiovisual materials—such as videos, slide-tape shows, and flip charts—visually portray key messages during interpersonal communication sessions.

The rules for selecting channels are basic but very important:

1. Select channels that reflect the patterns of use of the specific target audience, not the tastes of the communication team or decision makers. Almost all communicators have their "favorite media," whether video, puppets, or radio. In order to have an impact, however, the channels selected must be those that "reach" their target audience with the greatest degree of frequency, effectiveness, and credibility.
2. Recognize that the different channels play different roles.
3. Use several channels simultaneously. The integrated use of multiple channels increases the coverage, frequency, and effectiveness of communication messages.
4. Select media that are within the program's human and financial resources.
5. Select channels that are accessible and appropriate to the target audience. Radio messages should be scheduled for those radio stations that the target audience actually listens to and at broadcast times when that audience listens. Print materials should be used only for literate or semiliterate audiences who are accustomed to learning through written and visual materials. Materials should be distributed in accessible and visible places where the target audience already goes. Interpersonal communication should be provided reliably by credible sources (United States Department of Health and Human Services, 1989).

The combination of these channels is called the media mix. The media mix selected should be one that enables communicators to reach many people many times within the stipulated time frame, to supply the appropriate information in an understandable form for each target audience, and to remain within a budget that can be maintained by the institution conducting the communication program.

There are many excellent books written on how to select channels and how to develop, pretest, and use broadcast messages and print materials in developing countries. Several of these books are mentioned in the supplementary reading list at the end of the book. The following sections will discuss how a behavioral approach can strengthen the way channels are used within a behaviorally focused communication strategy.

Using Communication Channels as Consequences

Communication channels have commonly functioned as antecedents to target behaviors—providing information, teaching skills, and creating demand for products and services. However, communicators should also consider using these channels to strengthen the link between a target behavior and its consequences. Other behavioral theories also predict a strong behavior-consequence link, and social marketers look at benefits when promoting a product or behavior. Unlike these other theorists, however, communicators would strengthen the behavior-consequence link by continuing to rely on actual observed behavior rather than on mental interpretations of the relationship between behavior and consequences. The resulting strategy would use the channels to provide models of the behavior and its consequences. For example, radio and television spots can show people performing the behavior and experiencing certain consequences that would appeal to the target audience.

Communication channels might function as consequences in at least three ways.

Introducing a New Consequence for the Target Behavior

When a consequence is not immediately obvious because of the preventive nature of a behavior, communicators can introduce new positive consequences until more natural consequences are experienced. Print materials, such as diplomas and certificates, can reward compliance or mastery of skills; Ministry of Health newsletters can profile outstanding primary health care workers or effective health programs. Interpersonal channels help to create a supportive environment by providing positive feedback to primary audiences for their behavior; for example, a clinic worker can praise a mother for keeping her child on schedule for his immunizations. Mass media spots and programs can praise the primary audience for performing target behaviors. Radio and television spots can provide models who are correctly performing the target behaviors and are rewarded for performing them.

If the communication strategy introduces new consequences, communicators would also use communication channels to teach the individual to recognize the new consequences. Radio and television spots can inform audiences that rewards or diplomas are available for successfully completing a health practice and can motivate family members to reinforce target behaviors.

Lowering Negative Consequences

Communication channels also can be used to lower consequences for engaging in target behaviors. In some cases, the communicator cannot directly change the negative consequence itself but can reduce its impact on the target audience. For example, malaria prophylactics can cause side effects. Communication channels can provide information about those effects, teaching the target audience that they are normal and necessary for the medication to be effective.

Increasing the Saliency of Consequences

Child survival technologies and required behaviors are evolving. New behaviors generate new consequences. Communicators often need to increase the saliency of a relatively unknown consequence. Many people in the developing world simply did not know that the lack of vitamin A could cause night blindness. Communication strategies that focus on increasing the saliency of this consequence, however, would not necessarily produce recommended preventive behaviors, since only a few children actually get night blindness. Preventing this disease is not particularly salient to the target audience. Research is now demonstrating, however, that increased doses of vitamin A can lower the risk of death from other, more common childhood diseases. Communication channels can now promote a more meaningful consequence to parents. In most countries, broadcast channels are particularly effective in this role, since they can reach a large number of people in a short period of time.

Using Communication Channels in the A-B-C Chain

Table 4.1 illustrates the way channels might function to trigger, shape, and reward target behaviors, specifically considering the demographic and socioeconomic characteristics of developing country populations. The number 1 indicates that this channel would be particularly strong in this function. A 2 means that the channel would probably be fairly strong. A 3 indicates that this channel would probably be relatively weak in this function but could be used in conjunction with other channels. A blank means that this channel would probably not perform well in this function. The numbers in the table are intended to serve only as an example of one program's analysis of how to use communication channels. Communicators should come up with different ratings for their own target audience and selected health practices.

Table 4.1 is designed to help communicators visualize how the different channels could function within the A-B-C chain, but not to encourage them to select among the channels. Again, the question is not which channel is best but, rather, how these channels can be used in an integrated way to support and reinforce behavior of a specific target audience (United States Department of Health and Human Services, 1989).

Tables 4.2 and 4.3 illustrate ways in which the three channels—interpersonal, broadcast, and print—could be integrated to create an environment of support for mothers who are not completing the immunization schedule in an EPI program because of a skills deficit: approximations to target behaviors exist, but they are not being performed with sufficient frequency or at the right time. The EPI program objective is to increase the number of children with completed vaccination series. Communicators translate these objectives into the following target behaviors:

Table 4.1. The Role of Communication Channels in the A-B-C Chain.

Strategy	*Interpersonal*	*Broadcast (Radio/ Television)*	*Print*
Antecedents			
Increase knowledge	1	1	2
Create awareness or demand	2	1	2
Motivate trial	1	1	2
Give timely reminders	2	1	2
Practices			
Teach complex skills	1	3	2
Shape approximations	1	2	
Provide feedback	1		
Teach frequency	1	1	2
Teach duration	1	1	2
Teach accuracy	1	1	2
Teach timing	1	1	2
Consequences			
Decrease unpleasant consequences	1	2	
Introduce pleasant consequences	1	1	2
Increase the saliency of a consequence	1	1	3
Decrease rewards for competing or nondesired behavior	1	1	3

Mothers: (1) Bring children to the clinic at appropriate intervals for immunizations. (2) Bring the immunization card to every clinic visit, even if it is not immunization day.

Health workers: (1) Ask for and check the immunization card every time a mother brings her child to the clinic, even if it is not immunization day. (2) Bring the immunization series up date whenever a child is found to be behind schedule.

Table 4.2. Communication Strategies to Provide Antecedents and Consequences: Primary Audience—Mothers.

	Interpersonal	*Broadcast (Radio/ Television)*	*Print*
Antecedent	Schoolchildren inform neighbors of need for immunization and also tell them to bring vaccination card when they go. Church group has speaker present on EPI. Urges mothers to immunize their children and to take the vaccination card when they go.	Spots inform mothers of clinic schedule/immunization schedule. Spots tell/motivate mothers to bring vaccination card to clinic.	Posters urge mothers to seek immunizations and bring their immunization card. Vaccination calendar painted on billboard/clinic wall. EPI poster displayed at pharmacy.
Consequence	Nurse praises mother for coming on time. Nurse praises/thanks mother for bringing her vaccination card. Mother-in-law provides child care while mother is away at clinic. Women's co-op starts support group; mothers share experience with EPI.	Spot congratulates parents whose children are fully immunized News item about coverage rates achieved in town/region.	Diploma given for completed immunization series. Stickers put on immunization card for each visit.

Table 4.3. Communication Strategies to Provide Antecedents and Consequences: Primary Audience—Health Workers.

	Interpersonal	*Broadcast (Radio/ Television)*	*Print*
Antecedent	Health worker is trained in immunization skills. Supervisor reminds health worker to check card.	Health worker radio program reminds health worker to check vaccination card. Spots publicize outreach work of community volunteers.	National EPI policy is displayed in clinic sign. Poster on the refrigerator reminds health worker to check vaccination card. Special smock with writing or a picture on it is given worker to wear on immunization days.
Consequence	Supervisor observes health worker–mother interaction and praises health worker for checking card. Supervisor discusses coverage advances at regional meeting. Staff receive recognition. Monthly health worker meetings are held to discuss EPI progress/problems.	Clinics with high completion rates are mentioned on radio/television Spots highlight role of volunteer workers in raising coverage rates.	Clinic coverage is published in regional newsletter. Clinic coverage chart is displayed in the clinic. Certificate is given to health worker who brings the most children up to date in their immunizations.

Summary

Communicators plan for a behaviorally focused communication program by analyzing the relationships between the environment and the desired behaviors. They take those relationships into consideration when selecting target behaviors, planning communication strategies, and defining the role of communication channels. Specifically, this chapter provides a behavioral approach to selecting target behaviors that are most amenable to change and that have the most potential impact on the health problem; selecting and developing communication strategies that focus on skills and performance deficits by teaching and supporting skills development and creating an environment of support to maintain learned behaviors; and selecting integrated interpersonal, print, and broadcast channels to function as consequences as well as antecedents to target behaviors.

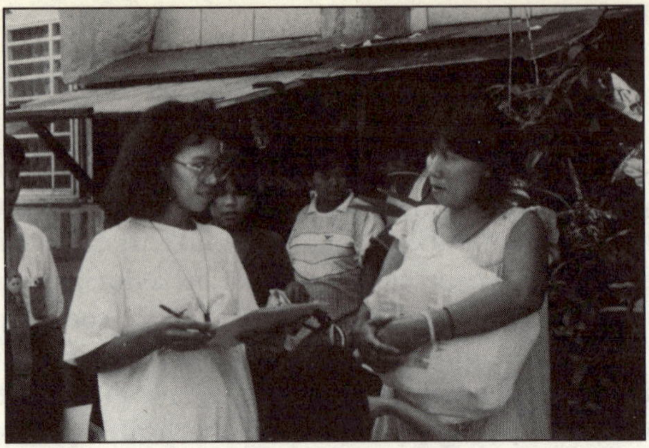

5

Skills Training

Training is a major activity during the implementation phase of a health communication program. During implementation, training becomes a partner with broadcast and other communication channels to strengthen skills necessary for building and maintaining behaviors critical in child survival programs. If training is being used as a strategy specifically for behavior change, then its primary focus will be on skills acquisition. This focus has implications for the techniques and instruments used in training.

Much of behavioral theory emphasizes remedies for performance deficits. For example, setting up effective cues for behavior or providing appropriate reinforcement can strengthen the "A-B" and the "B-C" relationships and thus make a behavior more likely to occur. But what if a person actually does not have the skills to perform a behavior? Enter training. The behavioral model of training described in this chapter places greater importance on skill development than on knowledge change, since a person who lacks skills cannot benefit from the most supportive of environments. Based heavily on social learning theory (Bandura, 1977), as well as applied behavior analysis (Baer, Wolf & Risley, 1968), this model assumes that a person needs practice with a skill or at least needs to observe others performing that skill in order to perform it him or herself. In skills training, communicators continue to focus on observable behavior. The specific skills needed, of course, will vary substantially according to disease-specific interventions, the goals of the public health program, and the target audience. For example, clinic staff are taught case management and interpersonal communication skills, while mothers are taught prevention and home treatment skills and the ability to recognize when they need to seek help from the medical system. All these practices rely on adequate skill levels, however; so skills training is necessary for all people involved in children's health.

Figure 5.1 shows a continuum of training opportunities that occur in public health programs. Skills-training methods can be used anywhere on this continuum, from highly specialized professional levels for supervisors and health care providers to the training of village health workers in one-on-one counseling of mothers.

One of the key roles health workers play in child survival is to communicate with mothers and teach them how to prevent and treat childhood illnesses. Health workers should see themselves as and be trained to be trainers of mothers as well as healers of sick children. Indeed, training is not only conducted in formal workshops or sessions but also takes place during any contact between health worker and mother and between supervisor and health worker.

Since health care providers are trainers as well as healers, they need to know *how* as well as *what* to train. People tend to teach other people in the same way they are taught. Health workers, therefore, should be trained in the same way that they will train mothers and with the same techniques they will use with mothers. When health workers counsel mothers, they are creating a training situation parallel to their own training. Although mothers' informational needs are different, the health worker can apply the same behavioral principles and training techniques to the counseling session. The five steps of skills training outlined in this chapter can be applied equally to the training of health workers and to the training of mothers.

Figure 5.1. Training and Feedback Loop.

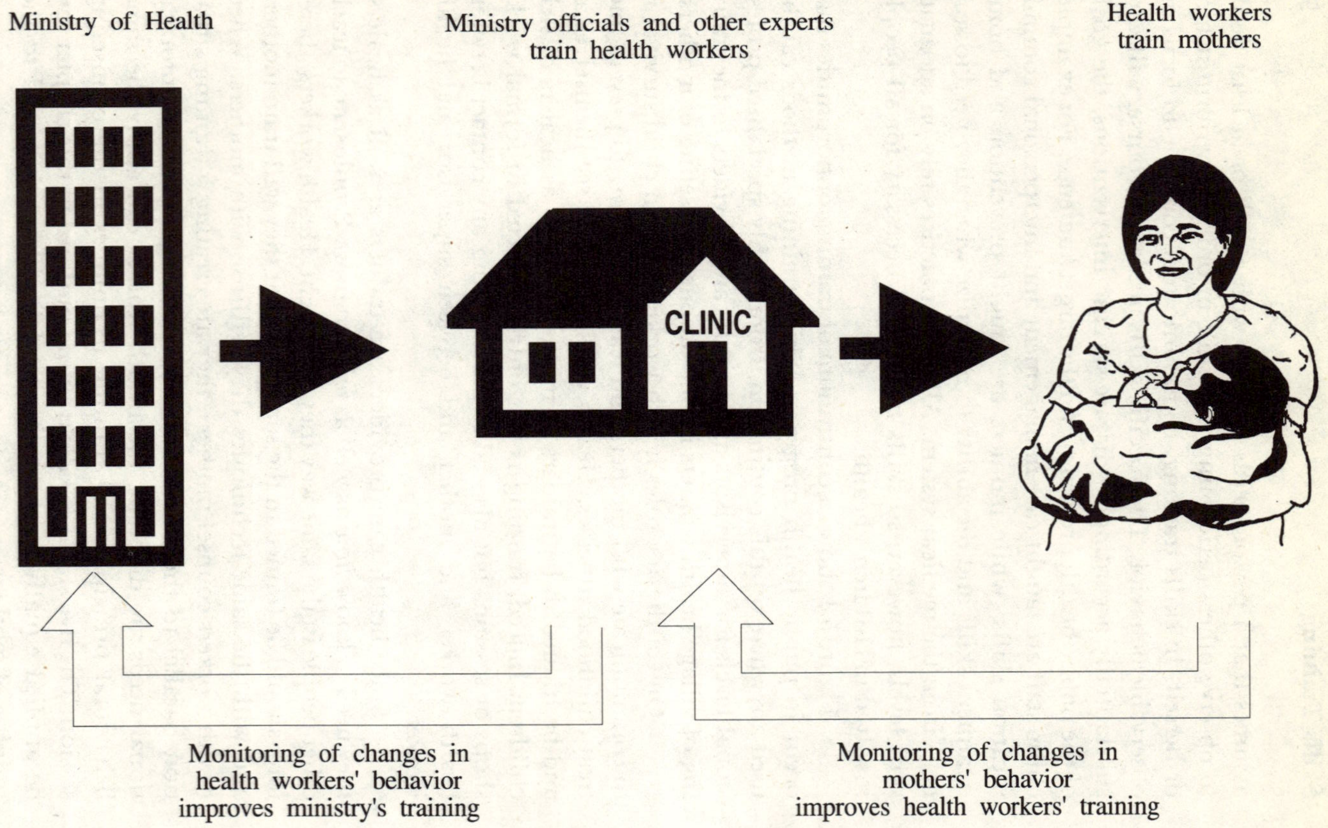

Using Behavioral Observation to Plan and Evaluate Training

The training of health workers usually covers areas such as basic diagnostic and treatment skills, effective health education, proper use of teaching aids, and methods of teaching mothers to use child survival technologies. In each case, training focuses on demonstrating and practicing the skills necessary to perform each of these tasks. Although surveys of trainees can be used to assess knowledge levels, their skill deficits can best be measured by direct observation. Just as communicators used observation to select mothers' target behaviors (Chapter Three), observations of actual (not reported) behavior can help communicators design the training curriculum by measuring the degree to which skills are present or lacking. Indeed, as illustrated in Figure 5.1, the actual behavior of people trained provides the most relevant guidance to the planning of training. The primary focus of the training is to build skills that have been observed to be weak or lacking.

The sequence of planning and evaluating training programs with behavioral observation is as follows:

1. To aid in structuring these observations, program planners list the behaviors deemed necessary to perform a specific skill—for example, the steps of mixing and administering ORS or giving a health talk.

2. Trained observers check off when and how frequently the desired behaviors occur. Before and after training, trainees are observed in natural situations or in role plays.

3. Results can be tallied in several different ways. For example, when health workers are being trained to conduct group health education sessions, an observer can tally the number of health workers correctly performing one particular teaching skill—probably before and certainly after the training. Program trainers can then determine what specific skill deficits need to be addressed and subsequently who benefited from training in that area. Each individual trainee's performance of all the skills needed for group health education sessions can also be graphed. Such a graph can show how an individual's skill level changes during training, or is maintained or deteriorates over time.

Exhibit 5.1 presents a checklist similar to that used to evaluate health workers in a recent HealthCom project in West Java, Indonesia. These health workers were given diarrhea counseling-cards and brief instructions in how to use them. One card showed the diagnostic algorithm for diarrhea; four color-coded cards described the appropriate recommended treatment for the mother to follow. The health volunteers then used the diagnostic card and one of the four treatment cards (depending on the severity of the diarrhea of the child whose mother they were counseling) in a role-play situation. Observers "rated" the performance of three health workers, using the checklist shown as Exhibit 5.1, and gave these data to the trainers so that they could determine what additional training needed to be conducted.

The data presented in Exhibit 5.1 show that the counseling cards worked well: the health workers made the right diagnoses and

Exhibit 5.1. Checklist for Evaluating Skills of Health Workers Counseling Mothers About Treatment for Children's Diarrhea.

Skill	Health Worker I		Health Worker II		Health Worker III	
	Yes	No	Yes	No	Yes	No
Listened to mother without interrupting	✓		✓			✓
Asked questions from diagnosis card	✓		✓		✓	
Made correct diagnosis	✓				✓	
Selected correct counseling card	✓		✓		✓	
Read directions	✓		✓		✓	
Showed mother how to mix ORS		✓	✓			✓
Showed mother how to administer ORS		✓	✓		✓	
Had mother practice these two steps	✓		✓			✓
Gave praise as was appropriate		✓		✓		✓

selected the corresponding treatment cards. But the health workers still needed more training in how to demonstrate mixing and give mothers praise. The trainers had the health workers practice these skills in their follow-up sessions, and two weeks later they evaluated the health workers again. This time, the role plays proceeded virtually flawlessly, indicating that the health workers not only knew how to use the counseling cards but also knew how to demonstrate mixing and reinforce mothers for trying out the skill (Exhibit 5.2).

The following example demonstrates how behavioral observation was used in a training workshop for health workers to learn how to counsel mothers of children with diarrhea.

Several health workers attended a two-day regional workshop on health education. At the beginning of the workshop, each participant was asked to demonstrate how he or she would conduct a clinic visit with a mother. In a brief three-minute simulation,

Exhibit 5.2. Checklist for Evaluating Health Workers' Skills After "Booster" Sessions.

Skill	Health Worker I		Health Worker II		Health Worker III	
	Yes	No	Yes	No	Yes	No
Listened to mother without interrupting	✓		✓		✓	
Asked questions from diagnosis card	✓		✓		✓	
Made correct diagnosis	✓		✓		✓	
Selected correct counseling card	✓		✓		✓	
Read directions	✓			✓	✓	
Showed mother how to mix ORS	✓		✓		✓	
Showed mother how to administer ORS	✓		✓		✓	
Had mother practice these two steps	✓		✓		✓	
Gave praise as was appropriate	✓		✓		✓	

trainers observed the quality of health workers' communication, using a female trainer or a local health professional to act as the "mother." From this exercise, trainers observed that nine out of ten trainees gave ORT instructions correctly, and six of ten demonstrated mixing. Two of the ten asked the "mother" to practice the mixing procedure; however, neither one gave feedback to the mother on how well her practice went. None of the health worker trainees used any open-ended questions in their brief session. These findings gave trainers a clear idea of where skill strengths and weaknesses lay.

Next, in preparation for the workshop, trainers wrote specific behavioral objectives specifying these three skills. The subsequent workshop focused on how to ask open-ended questions and on why and how health workers should use simulated practice and feedback when counseling mothers.

After the workshop, a final observation of the same type of simulated practice indicated improvement on all the skills. Of particular interest to the trainers was that the mean number of open-ended questions had risen from 0 to 2.2 per simulation. The trainers made a graph of each health worker's performance scores as a baseline, and then visited the health workers' clinics in the ensuing six months. In observing their interactions with mothers in the clinic, trainers again checked whether health workers used each of the skills practiced in training. They also graphed the number of open-ended questions the health workers asked. These field observations not only showed how well the trainees had maintained their skills but also provided the trainers with a needs assessment for future workshops.

To avoid making the training overcomplicated or oversimplified, the trainer must get some idea about the knowledge and experience level of the participants. When resources allow, there is no replacement for direct behavioral observations of existing skills as a needs assessment. If only a brief amount of time is available before training, however, a few open-ended questions concerning a certain skill are better than no assessment at all. Instead of assessing with simulations or on-site observations, for example, trainers may ask health workers the following questions:

"How many of you have given health talks (or "health talks on topic X")?"
"What techniques did you use?"
"What were the mothers' reactions?"
"Can you show me how you talk to mothers?"

Training can then be based on responses to these questions or on tallies of direct observations. For example, all skills necessary for effective face-to-face communication need to be included in training, but if evidence from assessment shows that trainees are already performing some skills fairly well, these skills could be reviewed briefly in training. On the other hand, if assessment shows that certain communication skills are not being performed or not being performed well, these need to be introduced and practiced in training. The same goes for content areas. Scores from assessment will indicate what information is accurately or inaccurately stated and what information is not mentioned at all in most health talks the trainees give. This will guide the trainer in what health information needs correcting and practice or simply needs reinforcement in training. In this way, training is customized to the needs of the trainees and makes the best use of precious training time.

Five Steps of Skills Training

Skills training consists of five essential steps: instructions, demonstration, simulated practice, feedback and reinforcement, and homework (practice assigned outside of training). Instructions and demonstrations are common to many formal educational situations and training formats. Skills are best learned, however, when repeated practice, feedback, and reinforcement occur in training. Without mastery in training, it is unlikely that the skills will be used in real-life situations. The steps of practice, feedback, and homework, then, are most important in achieving behavior change through training.

Step 1: Instructions

Instructions are similar to didactic teaching, whereby knowledge about general skills and component behaviors is transmitted. This step, although necessary, should play only a minor introductory role in the skill development process. Effective instructions serve only as preparation (an antecedent) for skills development and cannot replace behavioral practice in the learning process. Instructions generally include a description of the skill, specifying action to be taken rather than knowledge to convey or attitudes to portray. For example, "Greets mothers and asks how they are" is a clear instruction of what to do, whereas "Shows respect for mothers" is not.

Instructions also can include the rationale for using a skill. In the training of health workers, a rationale for asking mothers about their current practices before giving instructions for home care is "You ask a mother about her current practices first so that you can fit your messages to her demonstrated skill and knowledge level."

As important as what is *said* during the instructional phase is how well it is *understood.* Trainers need to assess to what degree the trainees understood the information. Often they conclude instructions with a close-ended "Do you understand" or "Was it clear"—to which participants nod their heads affirmatively. This strategy gives trainers little useful information about how well the audience truly understood the instructions. More useful information usually is elicited by open-ended questions about the topic and other forms of two-way communication between professional trainers and health workers or between health workers and mothers. For example, the question "What is your husband's reaction to your breast feeding?" is likely to yield much more useful information than "Does your husband approve of breast feeding?" Questions that begin with "how" or "what" are preferable to those that require a simple "yes or no" response.

By using this type of instructional approach (in other words, setting up a dialogue about a topic), the trainer establishes a more personalized type of communication and a feeling of openness about the message. Through two-way communication, trainers also gain direct evidence about their effectiveness as communicators. If a trainee is not able to state important parts of the message correctly, the instructions themselves should be reexamined. Perhaps the vocabulary is inappropriate, too much information was given too rapidly, more concrete examples should be given, and so on.

Step 2: Demonstration

In the demonstration phase, the trainer demonstrates the target skill and further ensures that the participants fully understand the instructions that have been given. Demonstrations help clarify the verbal description of the component behaviors. Such clarification is especially important when the language or manner of speech of the trainer and trainee is different—for example, when a health worker and mother are from different regions or ethnic groups. Demonstrations are also important when target skills are relatively complex—for example, when health workers are learning to fill out a child's immunization or growth-monitoring card or combining effective case management with counseling in a clinic visit.

The trainer does not necessarily need to be the model. In cultures where such a process would be appropriate, participants can learn from observing one another performing the behavior. The trainer, however, should select a demonstrator who is known to be fairly good at the skill and who would not be criticized by others for "putting on airs." The model does not always have to be present. If a woman in the village is well known but is not participating in the present health education session, that woman can still be referred to in the third person, so that mothers can think back on what she does to keep her child healthy. During the demonstration session, the trainer can point out which aspects of the third-person model's behavior are most important. In such cases, the trainer again needs to select a well-respected woman who would not suffer for having been held up as an exemplar. Also, the trainer must be very specific about the behavior to be imitated, so that the trainees do not learn the wrong lesson.

Case Study: Use of Modeling in an
ORT Campaign in Papua New Guinea

A novel approach to modeling was included as part of an ORT campaign in Papua New Guinea, which had the luxury of placing VCRs and televisions in central health centers where health workers came to pick up their paychecks every month. A training video for the workers, entitled *Making Things Clear,* was produced and distributed to these centers, where the health workers were encouraged to watch it during their visits. The video began with a rationale for effective interpersonal communication, after which the narrator announced that they would watch a scene of how not to communicate. In this scene, a health worker is depicted as rushing a mother through a clinic visit, treating her brusquely, using highly technical language, and failing to include modeling or other behavioral training steps. In the next scene, the model demonstrates the skills necessary for more effective counseling. The narrator's review of the critical steps in "making things clear" concludes this innovative video.

Step 3: Practice

Practice is performance of the behavior in the presence of the trainer. This is the only way to ensure that trainees really master the targeted skills and are able to do them on their own after training.

In the practice sessions, as many of the trainees as possible try target skills. They may simply repeat the component behaviors, or they may simulate real-life situations in a role play. After the training sessions are over, practice continues in the trainees' workplace or home. (This homework is discussed later as Step 5 of the skills-training process.)

Practice in the training sessions should be set up to resemble the real-life situations participants will face later. For example, when health workers train mothers, many of whom will have their babies with them, the babies can be incorporated into the practice session to make it more realistic. Mothers can go through an entire sequence of mixing ORS and even administering a spoonful of the solution to their babies in the training session. In this way, the health worker will know for certain that the mother is capable of carrying out the prescribed task. When health workers are the trainees, they may take turns playing "mothers" in order to make their practice of health talks or demonstrations as realistic as possible.

Practicing a skill once in training greatly helps trainees move from knowing about a skill to being able to do it. Practicing the skill several times in training allows them to go further and become fluent in the skill. With *repeated* practice and feedback in training, trainees leave the session better able to perform the task in their workplace or home and are less likely to lose the skill level they achieved in training. Training sessions and workshops are often overloaded with topics to cover, and actual practice time is one of the first segments to be cut. Yet, in the long run, if the agenda must be cut it would be better to allow time for trainees to master one or two skills in training than to be exposed to more "facts." Furthermore, trainers are often confronted with large groups of trainees, so it may not be possible for each trainee to practice every skill multiple times. In such cases, practice should continue until the trainer sees that adequate "vicarious learning" (learning by watching others) is taking place (Bandura, 1977)—that is, until several consecutive participants show little or no difficulty in performing the new skill. Additional practice at this point may actually be boring.

Step 4: Feedback and Reinforcement

Feedback is information given to individual participants about the quality of their performance. If properly given, feedback will function as reinforcement by encouraging the participant to try the new behavior again, with specific strategies on how to improve. To be effective as reinforcement, feedback must be specific, constructive, and pleasant. Positive feedback must give the trainees a clear idea of what behaviors they were doing correctly, so that they can repeat those behaviors. Negative feedback must make clear how trainees can correct behaviors they were performing incorrectly, and it should not overwhelm them by enumerating too many expected changes at one time.

The critical dimensions of feedback are *who* can give it, *what* behaviors should be reinforced or corrected, and *how* they should be reinforced. In addition to providing feedback themselves, trainers should solicit feedback from the other group participants and from the individual trainee. This procedure not only broadens the scope of feedback but gives everyone the opportunity to practice giving constructive feedback.

When selecting what skills or behaviors to reinforce, we need to remember that optimal skill levels are developed through successive behavioral trials and feedback experiences. In other words, individuals enhance skills by actually performing them and receiving response-specific feedback in order to eliminate ineffective behaviors and repeat the effective ones. Practice does not "make perfect" unless it is combined with feedback. Thus, trainees must be given constructive and encouraging feedback for behaviors that get closer and closer to a desired skill: "Catch them doing something right and reinforce them."

The criteria for giving reinforcing feedback will depend on the individual's current level of proficiency at the given task. When trainers have observed a person's initial performance level, they can define the criterion for reinforcing improved performance. Beginners, for example, should earn verbal approval for any improvement, even if the outcome is only a small step toward achieving the final goal. The initial tasks for beginners should be made relatively easy and short, so that they experience success and reinforcing feedback right away. As the trainee gets more proficient at the task, the task can be made more difficult, and the standard for earning reinforcement raised.

Trainers and participants alike need to learn how to be as constructive as possible in their feedback. Constructive feedback should be specific with respect to the skill (for example, "I noticed that you showed the mother how to spoon solution into her baby's mouth before having her do it") rather than being overgeneral ("That was well done"). When feedback is specific, the participant learns exactly what she did that was effective or what she can do differently the next time (for example, "Next time, *ask* the mother when she must return for another vaccination rather then *tell* her"). Rewarding feedback should be as specific as correcting feedback: "I was pleased to see that you ask each mother what foods she was using to wean her child" is potentially more effective than "Your growth-monitoring sessions are going well."

After the trainer has demonstrated the method of giving feedback participants themselves should use the same feedback methods when they watch others do a role play. The participants should state specific strengths they observed and should give suggestions for what can be changed. Finally, the trainer should give participants feedback on how well *they* gave feedback.

The following characteristics (adapted with permission from Geller, Lehman, & Kalsher, 1989) are essential for constructive feedback:

- Both reinforcing and correcting feedback should be specific and relate directly to observable behavior.
- The feedback should be timely, following the target behavior as closely as possible.
- Participants should be given a chance to respond to the feedback, and the trainer should be a "good listener" during this reaction.
- Trainers should give correcting feedback in a manner that avoids embarrassment to the participant.
- Trainers should present correcting feedback in the form of "what you can do differently next time," without suggesting that all problems must be solved in the first run-through. Trainers should remember to *shape* the behavior *one step at a time.*
- Trainers should end their feedback with words of encouragement, reaffirming approval of the performance and the expectation that such improvement in performance will continue. An additional "good job" from the trainer can be very important in ensuring that the trainee maintains the skill over a long period of time, and even in prompting him or her to teach the skills to others.
- At the end of the feedback, the participants should restate specific behaviors they will perform the next time they practice the skill.

Step 5: Homework

Homework with feedback is critical to maintaining the skills learned in training. Homework constitutes additional practice, similar to the practices done in training, that the trainees must perform outside the training session. For homework to be most effective in strengthening and maintaining learned skills, it must be checked by the trainer, and constructive feedback must be given; in other words, the behavior of carrying out a homework assignment (using new skills) must result in positive consequences, so that trainees will continue to use the skill in their own clinics or homes. The trainer should seek out opportunities to check homework assignments through occasional visits to local clinics or, if travel is logistically impossible, come up with creative ways to provide feedback to health workers newly emerging from training.

One possibility for follow-up is for health workers to learn how to give themselves feedback by self-monitoring, as described in Chapter Six. When they are given simple checklists and trained in direct observation, health workers can learn to monitor their own job performance. For example, health workers can keep track of the number of mothers who attend a health talk, participate verbally in the talk, and actually practice the skills being taught. Thus, health workers can continually and objectively attend to the critical lessons they learned during training without the immediate presence of a supervisor. To get feedback on the self-monitoring—critical for its use in skills maintenance—health workers can send their observation sheets to the trainer for written comments or save the sheets until either the trainer or health worker has the opportunity to travel.

Homework with feedback is also effective at other levels of training. Health workers can assign mothers homework after a counseling session in the clinic. For example, the mother may be asked to try using two packets of ORS over the next forty-eight hours, after which the health worker will check on progress during a home visit, give the mother constructive and encouraging feedback, and deliver a long-term supply of additional packets. If the mother is aware that someone cares enough to check up on her success or problems with this or any other health-related skill, she is much more likely to practice it.

To help mothers maintain the skills they have learned—especially if home visits are not possible—the health worker might ask the mother to demonstrate various aspects of the skill (for instance, the treatment of diarrhea) during subsequent clinic visits. This practice session, with feedback from the health worker, can serve as a valuable refresher session, because a mother whose child has not had a significant diarrhea episode for some time (for instance, six months) may have forgotten how to treat the condition.

Training as Reinforcement

Training, as it is typically designed, serves to prepare people for their work. In other words, it functions as an antecedent in the A-B-C chain. In this position, training can introduce new skills and begin the learning process, but as an antecedent, it is in a relatively weak position to maintain long-lasting skill development and behavior change. One can, however, shift training's function in a program to that of a consequence, so that it reinforces participants' learned behavior and contributes to skill enhancement and maintenance over the long term. This type of training session would focus less on basic skills acquisition and more on problem solving, practice, and feedback. These activities turn training into a tool for maintaining a trainee's performance over the long term. Follow-up training sessions might be incorporated into an already functioning general supervision or monitoring program if organizational structure, financial backing, and logistics are favorable. But whether called in-service training, continuing education, or group supervision, these follow-up sessions must be positive learning and motivational experiences for participants. In this way, training has become a positive consequence following behavior rather than an antecedent triggering behavior.

For training to act effectively as a consequence, the sessions should begin with trainees demonstrating how they have been performing skills learned previously. The trainer can then reinforce performance strengths and create a relevant agenda for the remainder of the session. Trainer and trainees alike contribute to reinforcing skill strengths and practicing remaining skill deficits. An imaginative administrator might have trainees "earn" new training opportunities through exemplary performance. For example, a nurse auxiliary who consistently follows up with mothers on ORS-mixing skills from a previous health talk might be sent to the district capital for a professional workshop.

Health workers training mothers can apply these same principles. First, in actual training, health workers should incorporate as many positive consequences into their sessions with mothers as possible. By asking mothers what they find reinforcing, health workers can make their health talks more rewarding to the mothers. For example, health workers might develop two or three different approaches to one health issue, according to the different experience levels of the mothers. Sessions for new mothers would emphasize learning and practicing basic knowledge and skills. Sessions with experienced mothers could emphasize problems encountered in applying child survival skills and suggestions for change. And over the long term, health education sessions themselves can provide positive consequences to experienced mothers by having them take important roles in the sessions. These women can explain or demonstrate procedures, lead a song or exercise, or describe their experience. Assuming this role might function as a positive consequence for those women.

A Training Sequence

Regional trainers working in a diarrheal disease control communication program prepared a series of workshops for groups of eight to ten nurses and nurse auxiliaries. Goals were set within the general area of improving face-to-face communication or counseling with mothers. Audiovisual and other materials were gathered, and logistical arrangements for the workshop were made.

Specific objectives emphasized (1) asking open-ended questions frequently and relatively more than close-ended questions; (2) checking for any skills deficits mothers may have and demonstrating correct performance of these skills; (3) having the mothers practice the skill (for instance, ORT) in the clinic; (4) providing constructive feedback to the mother; and (5) assigning homework.

In the first part of the session, trainers conducted a brief needs assessment by asking the participants about the methods they use to communicate with mothers. Trainers then gave a rationale for the training, which includes an emphasis on the importance of face-to-face communication and the limitations of any health promotion effort that does not include this aspect. They also defined open-ended questions, demonstration, practice, follow-up, and other target skills to the health workers. Each of these skills—both incorrect and correct versions—was modeled by the trainers, working in tandem with health workers who played the roles of mothers being counseled to use ORT. In the incorrect version, trainers made mistakes such as using close-ended questions and forgetting to do a demonstration. The participants were challenged to pick out the mistakes and give the trainers corrective feedback. The second time through, the trainers performed all steps correctly.

It was now the participants' turn to practice. First, in teams of three, they took turns counseling, with trainers in the role of mothers. During feedback, trainers and participants alike indicated what the "health worker" did well, what he or she could do differently next time, and how the "mother" felt during the session. In the next exercise, the remaining participants worked in teams of two to train groups of other trainees who pretended to be mothers attending health talks. After each practice segment, the trainers encouraged the participants to give one another constructive and specific feedback. The trainers, in turn, commented on their feedback techniques.

At the end of the training, the health workers left the workshop with two documents; a certificate of completion of the training and various checklists they can use to monitor their own behavior the next time they interact with mothers about diarrhea control. (For an example of such a checklist, see Resource A.) Over the next months, the regional trainers attempted to visit all alumni to review their progress on their homework and—when possible—to observe them training mothers.

Summary

This chapter presents ample information about how to conduct skills training. The information, when regarded in its entirety, may seem overwhelming. However, as discussed in this chapter, skills are not learned all at once. They must be broken down into small, manageable steps and shaped over time. Becoming a good trainer is such a skill. To begin to become effective skills trainers, communicators could break down the skills they would like to learn into small, manageable steps and then try those steps one by one. Trainers could start by selecting one of the steps they are particularly interested in—for example, constructing a checklist and using it to observe health talks. They then could add other skills one at a time until they are performing all the steps necessary for effective skills training. Correct health practices and effective communication involve many skills. Skills training, then, becomes an important component in most health communication programs. It is important for those working in the health system as well as for the primary target audience. Health workers, for example, should see themselves and be trained as *trainers* of mothers as well as *healers* of sick children.

By directly observing the skills covered in training, trainers learn the performance levels of trainees and are able to plan and evaluate training. Chapter Three describes observation techniques.

The five steps in skills training are instructions, demonstration of the target skill, practice, feedback, and homework with feedback. Ample time should be provided for practice and feedback in sessions, so that participants are actually able to perform the targeted skill when the training sessions are over.

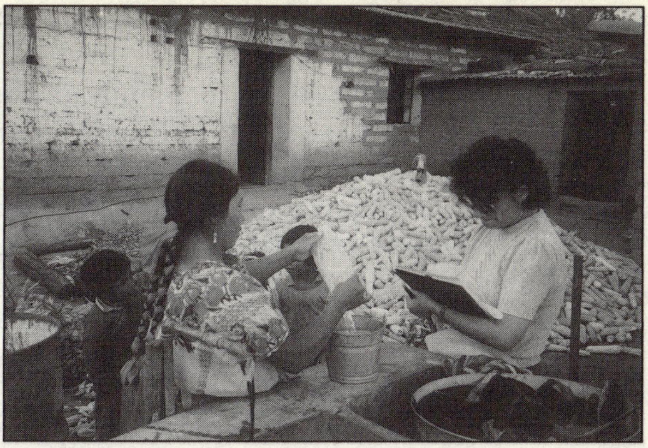

6

Monitoring Behavior Change

In the monitoring phase of a communication program, communicators continue their dialogue with the target audience. They use many of the same research techniques used in assessment to test the audience's reaction to the communication program and to measure the degree of behavior change achieved. They typically monitor *activities,* such as whether mass media spots are being broadcast according to schedule, how many health workers are being trained, and whether print materials are being distributed. They also monitor *reactions;* Did the members of the target audience hear the message and recall the information? This chapter, however, will focus on how to monitor *behavior change* and how data gathered from monitoring can be used to further change and support behavior. When communicators have specifically planned and implemented activities to change certain behaviors in a population, they need a methodology to determine whether any behavior change has occurred. This chapter will illustrate how a communicator can (1) use the same behavioral principles and methodology to design a monitoring system for measuring behavior change and (2) use the monitoring results to improve the communication program.

The goal of most health communication is to change behaviors so that people's health will ultimately improve. Communicators can evaluate the impact of their strategies by measuring changes in morbidity and mortality; yet the research needed to measure those changes is sometimes too expensive and time-consuming for a communication program to undertake. More important, it often takes years for changes in health practices to have a discernible impact on health statistics. Multiple factors—such as changes in living standards or legislation, war, and migration—influence trends in morbidity and mortality over time, so that even successful changes in health practices might get masked by other events. Despite the impact of multiple factors on health, most health professionals are convinced that certain critical behaviors, if widely practiced, would ultimately contribute to improved health status. The effectiveness of health communication can therefore be measured by the amount of change it has achieved in those behaviors.

Monitoring behavior change is based on two principles discussed in Chapter Two.

1. *Attitudes, beliefs, and knowledge can only be inferred from observations of what people do or say they do.* Communicators can demonstrate progress toward better health practices if they measure changes in a target population's actual behavior. People can change their behavior via many mechanisms: they can change attitudes or gain more information, or community norms can shift to make certain behaviors acceptable. It is difficult to measure reliably *how* people change, because this process is rarely observable to others or even perceptible to the people themselves. A communicator, therefore, in attempting to see how well a communication program is progressing toward its behavioral goals, should measure intermediate changes in *behavior* and not the mechanism by which people are changing. The methodology discussed in this chapter relies on directly observing behavior or quantifying indicators of behavior change.

2. *Behaviors are more likely to be repeated if they result in some type of positive consequence.* Communicators apply this principle in planning and implementation when they search for or create ways to reinforce target behavior. Reinforcement is also important for maintaining desired behavior over the long term. One

largely untapped source of reinforcement is the data collected from monitoring program participants' performance. As discussed in Chapter Five, feedback on performance can serve as a positive consequence and reinforce behaviors being performed. Thus, monitoring results themselves, if presented as feedback in a constructive and simple form, can help strengthen the very behaviors being measured. This feedback can be informal, as in the case of a health worker (the communicator) pointing out to the mother what she did correctly to treat her child's dehydration. Or it can be formal, as in the case of a trainer graphing four essential communication skills that trainees were practicing in a workshop so that the trainees can see from the graphs where their own performance needs extra work or is satisfactory.

In monitoring behavior change, communicators collect behavioral data, compile and graph results, and use the data as feedback to participants. Monitoring is therefore an effective tool in strengthening and maintaining behavior as well as in measuring behavior change.

Monitoring and Evaluation

A communication program can measure behavior change through both monitoring and evaluation. Sometimes monitoring and evaluation may actually measure the same behavior (such as mothers' skills in mixing ORS). In addition, many people refer to monitoring as process evaluation. This can cause confusion between the two procedures. The following section discusses the similarities and differences between monitoring and evaluation when they are used specifically to measure behavior change. Monitoring includes ongoing data collection of intermediate behavioral objectives, whereas evaluation includes data collection on the impact of health communication at some, often arbitrarily set, end date. Monitoring begins as soon as possible after a communication strategy is implemented and continues throughout. The communicator uses the monitoring data to help adjust the communication strategy and messages. Evaluation measures the impact of health communication after it has been in place for a period of time (frequently several years). Because evaluation data are collected infrequently, they cannot be used for feedback to a program as immediately or as frequently as can data from monitoring.

In monitoring, data are collected periodically, so that communicators can identify positive and negative trends as the program unfolds. In evaluation, data are generally collected twice: (1) before the communication strategy begins, to establish a baseline; and (2) after a period of several years, to create a postintervention comparison. As a safeguard against biasing the results, evaluation is often conducted by researchers not directly involved in the health communication activities. Although monitoring data also can be collected by outside researchers, they are most useful when they are collected, analyzed, and disseminated by the people who are actually involved in the communication activities.

Despite differences in purpose, some of the same methods are used in both monitoring and evaluation. Both procedures need to be designed so that data collected will credibly document that changes have occurred with exposure to the communication program. Usually, researchers create a comparison. One possibility is to collect data at two different times in the same location or with the same people (pre- and postintervention). Sometimes communicators have an opportunity to collect data before communication activities begin, thereby establishing a baseline from which later measures from the same location can be compared. Alternatively, data can be collected at the same time but in a geographical area outside the zone where the communication activities are occurring. This procedure enables the researchers to compare behaviors practiced by similar groups of people exposed or not exposed to the activities. In either case, the data collected can reveal to what extent behavior change was achieved with the communication program.

Communicators may use similar instruments in monitoring and evaluating behavior change, although some differences exist. Interview questionnaires probing a target audience's report of current practices are more commonly used in large, population-based, evaluation surveys; but program monitors also may want to conduct exit interviews—for instance, with mothers who have participated in a health education session at a clinic. Checklists, used to guide observation of target audiences' performance of selected behaviors, are particularly suited for monitoring; but such checklists also can

be used to validate verbal responses of a large evaluation survey with observational data from a subsample. Clinic records and product sale or distribution statistics are data sources useful to both monitoring and evaluating behavior change.

There is a vast literature on evaluation issues and methodology. Further reading is suggested at the end of the book. This chapter will focus on designing and carrying out monitoring of behavior change, and will not attempt to discuss other monitoring activities or evaluation because they are beyond the scope of this book.

Collecting Data for Monitoring

Because of the powerful impact feedback from monitoring behavioral data can have, it is important for the data to be collected in a suitable form. Program participants then can compile the data into a graph and immediately see what progress has been made on target behaviors.

Selecting Behaviors to Monitor

In order to decide what behaviors to monitor, program managers return to the list of core target behaviors selected in the planning stage. What communication activities have been tried, and what changes in target behavior can be detected following those activities? For example, one of the target behaviors in a diarrheal disease control program is mothers administering ORS in the home. Communication activities aimed at strengthening this practice might include training health workers to demonstrate mixing and administering ORS to mothers; making packets available to mothers from pharmacies, clinics, and community volunteers; and broadcasting radio spots to reinforce mothers' use of ORS during diarrhea.

To monitor changes in this behavior, communicators might measure individual health workers' demonstration and communication skills; number of packets distributed by source; and mothers' mixing and administration skills in the home. What is critical is that communicators are not monitoring an *activity* (How many participants were trained? How many clinics received posters and

brochures for mothers?); instead, communicators are monitoring progress toward the *behavioral objective* of the activity (How well can health workers demonstrate ORS mixing before and after training? Are mothers who have been given brochures treating common colds at home rather than coming to the clinic for antibiotics?). This focus gives communicators direct evidence of how much behavior change has been achieved. If monitoring these behaviors over time shows less than expected progress, communicators will want to improve the program strategy, design, or messages.

Monitoring Techniques

Several techniques are particularly well suited to monitoring behavior change. Three will be described here: direct observation, the use of clinical and other records, and self-monitoring.

Direct Observation. When complex behaviors—such as developing face-to-face communication skills, preparing and feeding a weaning food, and administering ORS—are being monitored, direct observation with a checklist provides useful data. The same procedures for accurate and reliable observation that were initially described in Chapter Three and applied to the design of training in Chapter Five would also apply when these behaviors are monitored. If the behaviors were observed in the assessment phase, the same instruments, observation procedure, and personnel can be used again in monitoring, to observe progress toward changing those behaviors. The amount of resources needed for monitoring will be minimized because the program has already developed necessary instruments and trained personnel in monitoring techniques. In addition, people are accustomed to being observed and are familiar themselves with the measurement instruments. Finally, when the same behaviors are measured over time with the same instruments and observers, any changes noted in behavior can be more readily attributed to program activities.

Clinical and Other Records. When less skill-dependent behaviors, such as timely immunizations and packet distribution are being monitored, clinical and other records can be useful. Monitoring

from records also indirectly measures many behaviors mothers do at home—for example, mothers' skill in recognizing signs of pneumonia and seeking medical help. The researcher can measure the mothers' behavior indirectly by comparing the number of pediatric pneumonia cases with the number of cases of common colds being brought to the clinic. Routinely kept clinic records have the advantage of providing a program with multiple data points and require little extra effort from staff, but monitors must also determine that these records present a reliable picture of what is actually occurring. One further advantage is that these types of records are fairly permanent, so the timing of data collection is more flexible.

Self-Monitoring. Anyone involved in the health of children might find self-monitoring a useful tool. Using this technique, individuals select behaviors of their own to observe, record their occurrence, and graph the results. Reading the graph itself gives them powerful feedback independent of others' biases. A mother determined to breast-feed might keep track of how many times or how long she breast-feeds her baby every day. A health worker may track how many times she greeted and praised mothers for being on time with the immunization series. In an urban clinic in Morocco and in a village health center in Senegal, nurses made and displayed graphs that reflect the number of prenatal exams they gave or immunizations they administered on a monthly basis. And clinic staff in Ecuador used pins stuck in maps to show which village households had fully immunized children and, implicitly, where more work was needed.

As with other monitoring activities, the data collected by self-monitoring can function as a powerful reinforcer of the behaviors being observed. The records kept during self-monitoring need to be graphed and displayed, so that the trends in behavior can be appreciated visually. The graphs can remain private or can be shared with an appropriate group such as colleagues or mothers.

Graphing Monitoring Data

The second step in monitoring behavior change is compiling and graphing the data. A graph is a picture of what is happening to an individual or a group of people over time. Graphing results allows participants to *see* changes and notice patterns of behavior that might emerge as time passes (such as fewer women coming to a clinic on market days or during planting season). Since one of the purposes of monitoring behavior change is to have the findings serve as feedback, portraying numerical data graphically allows people to visualize and easily understand changes.

Generally, any information can be graphed if it can be expressed as a number and can be collected at several points in time. Examples include graphing test results from training participants before and after training, the number of immunizations dispensed monthly, the number of health talks given and mothers in attendance, the number of outreach or home visits made weekly, the percentage of interpersonal skills a health worker uses with mothers, and the number of ORS packets the clinic dispenses monthly.

To make a graph, the monitor draws a vertical and horizontal axis. He or she labels the vertical axis to show what is being measured. Usually, this axis reflects the *quantity* of what is being measured, such as the number of questions a doctor asked, the amount a baby weighed, or the percentage of time a health worker talked in a group health lesson. Enough space must be left so that the results can be as high and as low as might be expected. Usually, the axis begins with zero at the bottom. (See Exhibit 6.1.)

Exhibit 6.1. Vertical Axis of a Graph.

(Quantity)	70
Number of	60
vaccines	50
given to	40
preschool	30
children at	20
clinic X	10
	0

Exhibit 6.2. Vertical and Horizontal Axes.

(Quantity)	70
Number of	60
vaccines	50
given to	40
preschool	30
children at	20
clinic X	10
	0

3/7 3/14 3/21 3/28 4/4 4/11

(Time)

The monitor then labels the horizontal axis to reflect time—that is, the date when the results were measured (daily, weekly, monthly), putting in specific dates and leaving sufficient space so that several measures can be clearly recorded. The more points on the graph, the more readily trends and patterns can be seen. (See Exhibit 6.2.)

The monitor plots the quantity that corresponds to the time it was gathered and then connects the dots or color in the bars (Exhibit 6.3).

After setting up a graph or a series of graphs, program monitors can simply enter data on a regular basis. After several data points have been recorded, the graphs are ready to be used as feedback.

Reinforcing and Maintaining Behavior Change with Monitoring Data

The third step in monitoring behavior change is using the results as feedback so that they reward and maintain desired behaviors. The data, now in graphic form, can serve as a powerful consequence in

Exhibit 6.3. A Completed Graph.

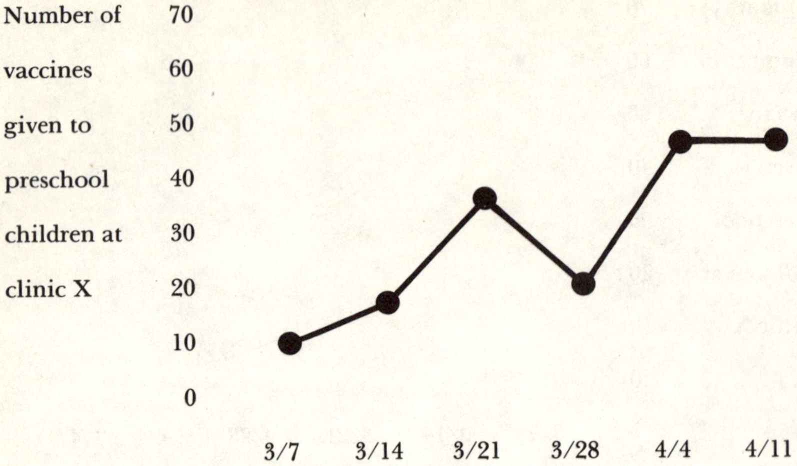

the form of constructive feedback to many participants in the communication program, from mothers to policy makers. Communication managers can highlight positive trends when reviewing data with program participants, return pooled data in graphic form to those who provided them, recognize health workers for improvements in performance illustrated by the monitoring data, and award certificates of achievement to clinics. By simply returning data in usable form, along with data from other clinics in the region, communicators enable health workers to make their own comparisons and reduce the sense of isolation that discourages them from maintaining satisfactory performance.

The following are four illustrative examples, compiled from a composite of field experiences, of how communicators can collect behavioral data, graph them, and then use them to provide constructive feedback to program participants.

Monitoring Health Center Utilization

The head of Mumba Clinic in a republic in central Africa made the graph shown as Figure 6.1, which tracks the number of immunizations her staff administered monthly at the clinic over a two-year

Figure 6.1. Number of Childhood Immunizations Given at Mumba Clinic, 1990–1992.

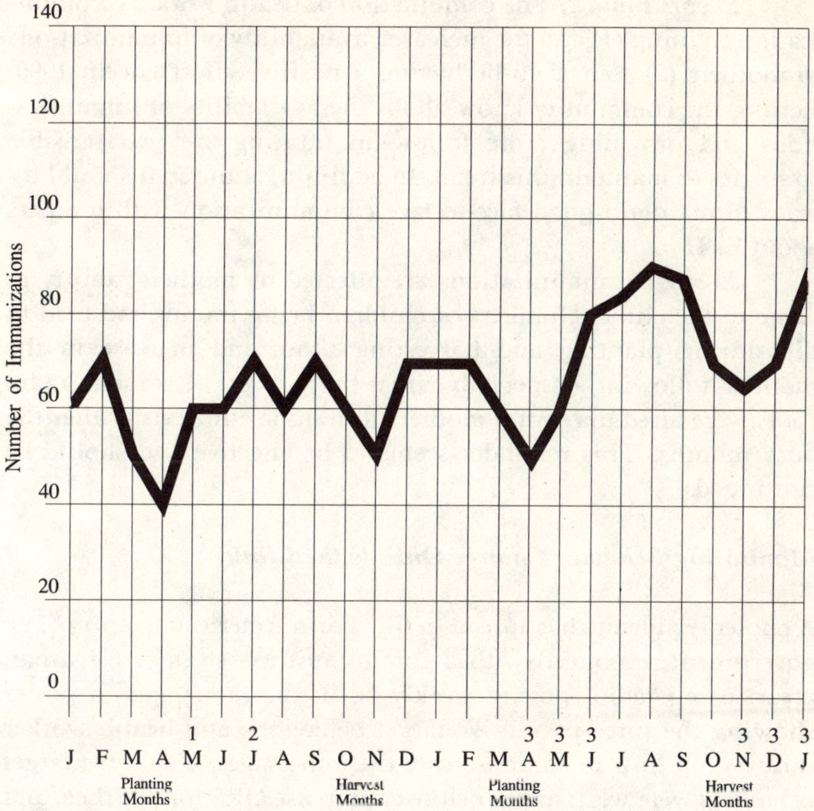

Key:

1 Health worker training in face-to-face communication skills.
2 Clinic refrigerators repaired, more immunizations available (donor assures supply).
3 Time and location for childhood immunizations aired on radio.

period. She took the data from the regular clinic records, made the graph, and then showed it to the staff for discussion.

The staff looked at the rise and fall of immunizations over two years, when health worker training in face-to-face communication and radio spots occurred, and drew the following conclusions about the effects of their communication program on demand for immunizations:

Events 1 and 2. The combination of health worker communication training (1) and the increased availability of immunizations to mothers (2) seemed to be having a positive effect late in 1990. Letting the community know about the availability of immunizations and providing more follow-up training are two possible strategies to maintain this trend. In addition, clinic staff should try ways to maintain good face-to-face communication with mothers about EPI.

Event 3. Immunizations are affected by mothers' ability to come to the clinic. Numbers of children being immunized tend to dip during planting and harvesting times and increase in the months following—especially after the harvest. Regional radio spots were aired to remind mothers to resume clinic visits after the busy months. This reminder seems to be effective and should be continued.

Monitoring Behavior Change Outside the Clinic

A cholera epidemic has spread to this Latin American country. The government responded with a communication strategy for urban areas, using radio spots, a weekly ad in the newspaper, a poster showing the three preventive target behaviors, and health worker training on how to communicate these messages. The three target behaviors were wash hands before eating, use ORS for diarrhea, and use latrines.

The Ministry of Health (MOH) team responsible for this communication program had three health promoters from local clinics go to three lunch counters, typically found at the edge of large markets, in order to observe hand washing among the clients. A fourth health promoter rotated among the three lunch counters to check the reliability of observations. These establishments usually provide a sink, water, and towel in the eating area to their clients. While eating lunch at the counter themselves, the monitors simply counted the number of clients served in an hour and noted how many of them washed their hands before eating. The monitors observed in lunch counters twice a week for seven weeks. Their data were converted to percentages (number washing hands over total number of clients) and then entered in the graph shown as Figure 6.2. The graph was presented at a meeting of health promoters and local health officials, the manager for the diarrheal disease control program, and health education unit staff from the central MOH, as well as the director of the radio station and the newspaper editor. They drew the following conclusions and made the following changes in the program from looking at the graph:

- The present communication strategy had the desired effect on target behavior, but it was still not at an acceptable level.

Figure 6.2. Percentage of Clients Washing Hands Before Eating at Three Lunch Counters near La Plaza Market (Phase I).

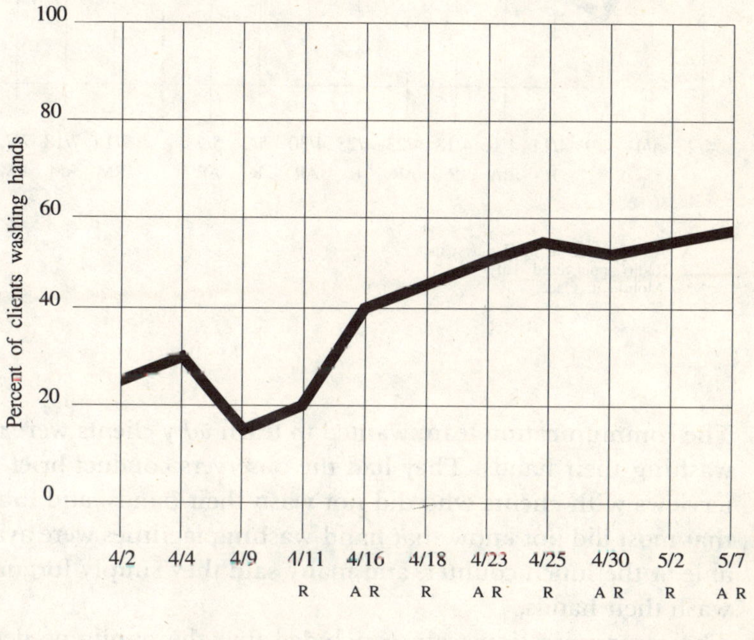

Key:
A Ad appeared in local newspaper.
R Radio spots aired daily.

Figure 6.3. Percentage of Clients Washing Hands Before Eating at Three Lunch Counters near La Plaza Market (Phase II).

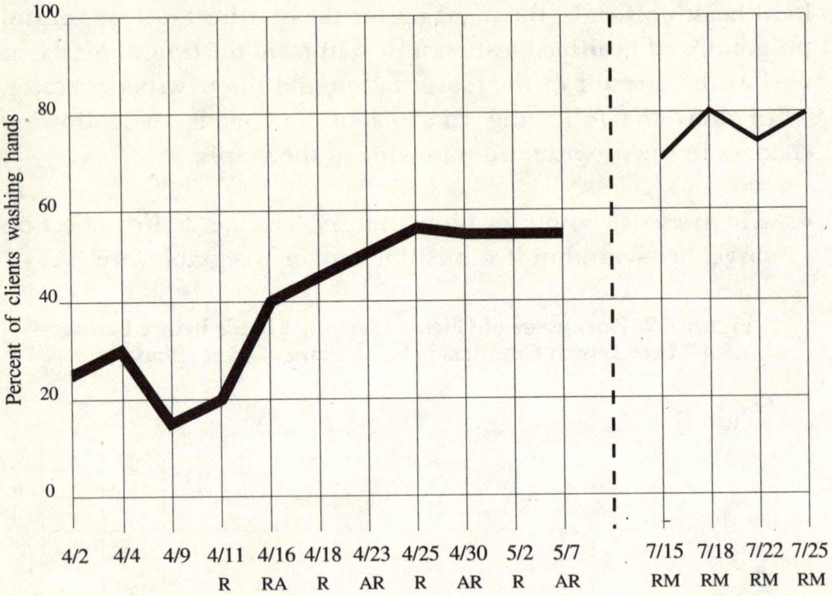

Key:
A Ad appeared in local newspaper.
R Radio spots aired daily.
M Mobile in place.

- The communication team wanted to learn *why* clients were not washing their hands. They had the observers conduct brief interviews with clients who did not wash their hands, and found that most did not know that hand-washing facilities were available at the lunch counter, and many said they simply forgot to wash their hands.
- The communication team concluded that the public needed a reminder at the time and place that hand washing was to occur. They produced an eye-catching mobile, reflecting themes already familiar to the public from the media. It was placed in the lunch counters over the hand-washing facilities. The mobile

served both to indicate that facilities were available and to act as a hand-washing reminder.

The graph shown as Figure 6.3 was produced from observations made after the mobile was in place and radio spots resumed. The observations indicated that the new communication strategy was indeed having an impact on the target behavior. The MOH team decided to continue the strategy and use the observations to measure whether the trend was maintained. They also decided to develop radio spots to inform the public of the results of the observations and praise them for performing this healthy practice.

Monitoring Training Outcomes

In an effort to decentralize health communication in this African country, the MOH trained regional clinic supervisors in health communication and training skills. The supervisors began their regional programs by training health workers in group communication skills, since many clinic-based health workers frequently conducted health talks with groups of mothers.

The supervisors selected fourteen health workers most responsible for health education in the region. They drew up a checklist of ten essential messages to be conveyed in diarrheal disease control and of twelve teaching techniques health workers should use when leading group sessions with mothers.

In September, the supervisors notified the health workers of the October training, showed them the checklists, and then observed them giving their usual group health talk in the clinic. They showed the checklists to the health workers, to help lower their anxiety about being observed by their supervisor. The supervisors also explained to the health workers that, since this was the first training activity, these observations were not a "test" but were designed to help the supervisors plan and evaluate the upcoming training. Since this was the first training these supervisors were conducting, they wanted to follow closely the performance of their trainees.

After conducting the training, the supervisors informed the health workers that they would be observed again giving group talks in the clinic. The supervisors used the same checklists as before and were able to make three observations over a three-month period following training. They graphed the results in several ways and used them as the focal point for a follow-up meeting held with the fourteen health workers. Two of the graphs are shown here (Figure 6.4 and Figure 6.5).

As shown in Figure 6.4, the average number of messages covered increased from five items before training to nine items afterward. That finding suggests that health workers learned the content of the messages in training. Over time, however, this per-

Figure 6.4. Average Number of Diarrheal Disease Control Messages Fourteen Health Workers Used in Health Talks Pre/Post Training.

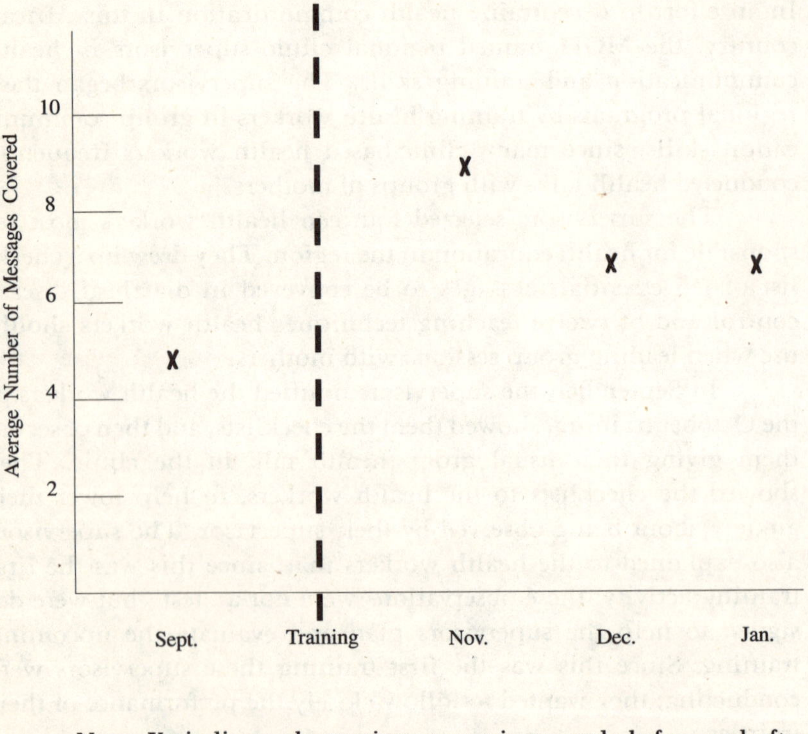

Note: Xs indicate observations supervisors made before and after training.

formance slipped to only seven messages on average being covered in actual clinic talks. Health workers found talks on diarrheal disease control complicated and usually "forgot" some of the key messages. The group therefore decided to make a reminder sheet that health workers could attach to the wall or place on the table in front of them when conducting group sessions.

As shown in Figure 6.5, the average number of communication skills increased just after training, from three to seven. However, absolute level achieved was unsatisfactory and decreased over time. Most of the skills focused on maximizing the participation of mothers during a session, an approach the health workers had never before experienced. The health workers felt that the skills of con-

Figure 6.5. Average Number of Communication Skills Fourteen Health Workers Used in Health Talks Pre/Post Training.

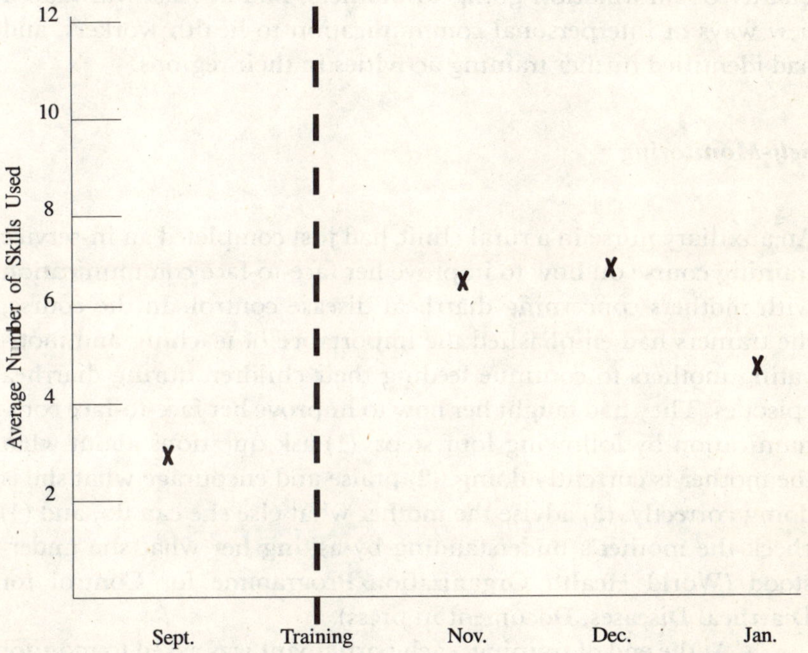

Note: Xs indicate observations supervisors made before and after training.

ducting a demonstration of mixing ORS and engaging mothers in the demonstrations were difficult to master, even though they had practiced these skills once in training. The health workers also felt that the participatory approach took too much time and they preferred just telling the mothers about treating diarrhea.

The trainers were struck by how much harder it was to change behaviors (communication skills) than knowledge (content items). They scheduled a follow-up training for the fourteen health workers to practice conducting mixing demonstrations and involving mothers in the sessions. They also decided that further training for new health workers in the region should include much more time for practice and feedback on conducting group sessions regardless of the health topic.

In general, the supervisors were pleased with the message from the graphs: they had made significant improvements in the quality of information going to mothers, had at least introduced new ways of interpersonal communication to health workers, and had identified further training activities in their regions.

Self-Monitoring

An auxiliary nurse in a rural clinic had just completed an in-service training course on how to improve her face-to-face communication with mothers concerning diarrheal disease control. In the course, the trainers had emphasized the importance of teaching and motivating mothers to continue feeding their children during diarrhea episodes. They had taught her how to improve her face-to-face communication by following four steps: (1) ask questions about what the mother is currently doing, (2) praise and encourage what she is doing correctly, (3) advise the mother what else she can do, and (4) check the mother's understanding by asking her what she understood (World Health Organization/Programme for Control for Diarrheal Diseases, Document in press).

At the end of training, each participant was asked to monitor how well he or she was putting these steps into practice. So the auxiliary nurse decided to try this self-monitoring exercise in her rural clinic. For the first three to four mothers she saw each day who had brought a child with diarrhea to the clinic, she marked on a piece of paper which of the communication steps she had performed. After a week, she made the graph shown as Figure 6.6.

The nurse found that during the first week (August 3 and 4), she had been quite conscientious about performing the four steps, but after the weekend she had reverted simply to giving advice without asking what the mother was already doing, without praising her, and without making sure that she understood the advice. The nurse was beginning to see that, despite *wanting* to use these effective communication methods she had learned in training, she was just too busy to use the four steps consistently. The nurse decided to try a visual reminder to help her remember to follow all four steps when she was communicating with mothers. She made a bright poster containing the four steps and placed it where she would see it when she was talking with mothers.

Figure 6.6. Example of Self-Monitoring.

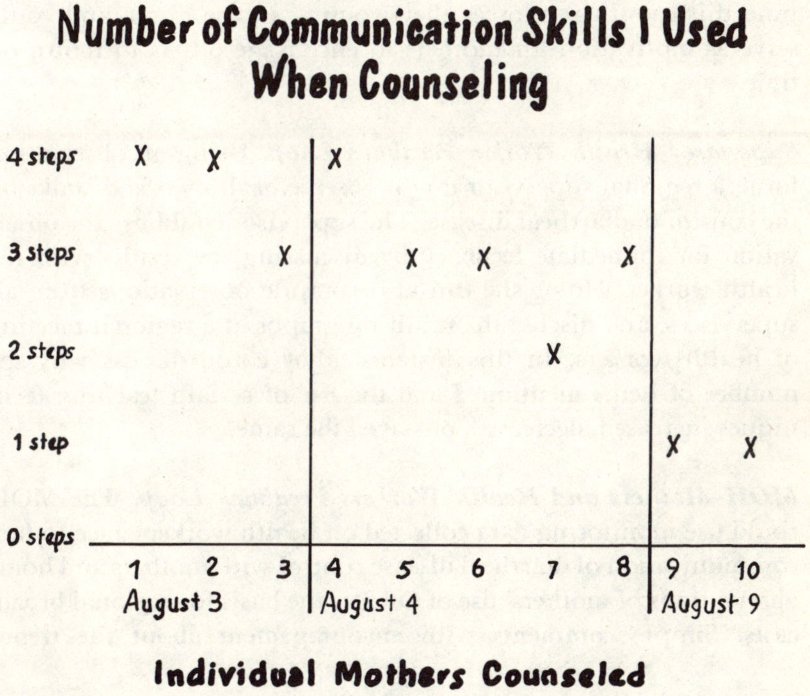

Creating Feedback Loops

The examples above illustrate how graphed results are used as feedback. They help program participants understand how and to what extent their communication, managerial, or outreach efforts have contributed to behavior change. They also show participants where they can make further improvements in their own behavior as well as in the communication program. These results can supplement formal mid-term or end-of-project evaluations to keep policy makers and donors abreast of the project's progress. The following are more examples of possible feedback loops that could be set up to strengthen and maintain behaviors.

Health Worker–Mother Feedback Loop. A health worker might keep track of how many mothers in the clinic's catchment area are on time or late for their infant's immunizations. The health worker could graph monthly totals and display them in the clinic. The graph itself serves as reinforcement for the health worker's efforts. Telling the mothers that more or fewer of their neighbors are on time this month reinforces their coming to the clinic and could serve as motivation for mothers to encourage others to return on time.

Supervisor–Health Worker Feedback Loop. Using an observation form, a regional supervisor might observe health workers' talks on the control of diarrheal disease. The supervisor could use the observation for immediate feedback by discussing the results with the health worker. He or she can also compile observations from all supervisees, and discuss the resulting graphs at a regional meeting of health workers. In this instance, they could discuss why the number of items mentioned and the use of certain teaching techniques increased, decreased, or stayed the same.

MOH–Mothers and Health Workers Feedback Loop. The MOH could use monitoring data collected on health workers' face-to-face communication of diarrheal disease control with mothers and home observations of mothers' use of ORS as the basis for regional broadcasts. Simple comments with encouragement about the trends shown on the graph in ORS usage in homes and the health workers' contributions could serve as a positive consequence from the MOH to health workers and mothers alike.

Treating Monitoring as a Behavior

Many communication program managers find it difficult to make monitoring systems work. Health workers are usually required to keep detailed records and to send reports to their supervisor. These activities are time-consuming and usually produce no feedback at all. In addition, the health worker is often criticized for being late or for reporting low levels of activity. Monitoring activities that take time and effort to do—keeping records, compiling data, sending reports to one's superior—meet either with no consequences at all or with punishment. These conditions cause monitoring behaviors themselves to change (health workers make up data to avoid criticism, reports come in late or are incomplete), or the monitoring system itself gradually weakens and eventually ceases to function. It is important, then, for participants to receive feedback from their monitoring, so that it is a positive, nonthreatening experience that helps their professional growth.

As with any behavior, monitoring behaviors can be trained, shaped, and supported. If monitoring is not currently practiced, communicators should break monitoring down into small steps and introduce one step at a time. For instance, they could select one communication activity that has clearly defined beginning and end points, can be observed, and is of immediate interest to participants, such as the health worker training described earlier in this chapter. In a few months, trainers would have feedback on the impact of their training and also would have a positive experience from monitoring their own program. As a result, these trainers/supervisors will be more likely to try monitoring other activities and to continue monitoring this one.

Other possibilities of introducing monitoring step by step are to take measures monthly instead of weekly, take one pre and one post measure instead of several, or take a few post measures if there was no opportunity to measure before an activity began. The important element is to make sure that measurement results are made visible to individuals involved in any way in an activity.

Summary

Communication programs that have set behavior change goals must monitor the progress being made toward those goals. Monitoring for behavior change involves three steps: collecting behavioral data, compiling and graphing the results, and using the data as feedback to participants. By performing all three steps, communicators can not only measure behavior change but also use the results as constructive feedback to strengthen the behaviors measured.

Measuring behavior change relies on the same instruments that were developed during planning or training. Findings are expressed quantitatively—the frequency or duration of target behaviors can be counted or measured. When these findings are graphed, participants can see improvements or weaknesses in their own behavior or in the behavior of others who are affected by a communication program. In addition, the reinforcing feedback of behavioral monitoring can be helpful in maintaining behavior change.

7

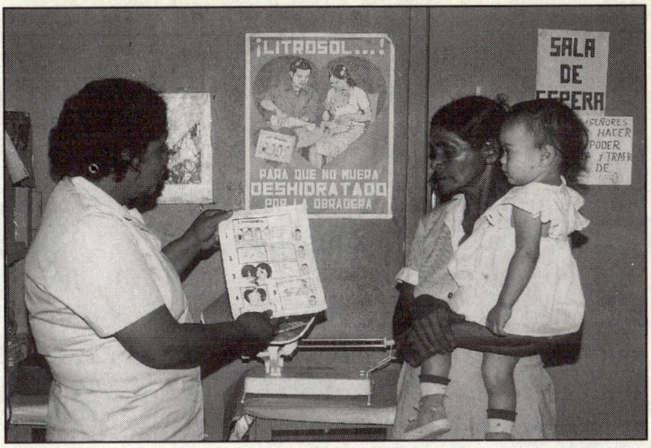

Maintaining Health Practices

A mother may have successfully completed the immunization series for her first child because, at that time, health workers were telling women about immunizations, mass media kept the schedule foremost in her mind, and vaccines were readily available. Two years later, she delivers another child. If supplies are now sporadic and the media spots have stopped, what in her social environment and in the immunization process itself will make it likely that she will repeat the series? Does she believe that her older child is healthy because he has been fully immunized? What are health workers doing at the clinic to encourage her to return? Are her neighbors immunizing their children? Is anyone in the family or neighborhood encouraging her as well? Are immunizations even mentioned on the radio? Is anything occurring to ensure that future mothers—younger sisters, nieces, and daughters—also have an opportunity to learn about and utilize immunization services? Without an environment of support for immunization practices, it is unlikely that this mother and new mothers will complete the series for their children.

Much effort and many resources have gone into designing and implementing communication programs to introduce behavior change in a target audience. Yet experience has shown that sustaining these changes over time is critical to making a meaningful public health impact. Until recently, however, ministries, donors, and communication planners have mostly responded to the need to introduce new health practices, such as ORT, growth monitoring, and vitamin A promotion. As a result, few resources have been allocated specifically to designing the communication programs to maintain learned behaviors over the long term. It is not surprising, then, after an initial project has been successful, to see a steady decay of program-induced changes in many health practices. Simply funding for longer periods the projects that successfully initiated changes is not the answer. Behavioral conditions necessary to foster the learning of new behavior are not necessarily the most favorable (or practical) conditions for long-term maintenance. Communication programs focusing on maintenance may therefore differ in message content and choice of primary audience, target behaviors, and communication channels. This chapter uses principles from behavior analysis to help communicators identify, plan, and implement programs that focus on maintaining the use of learned behaviors.

The tone of this chapter will necessarily be different from that of other chapters. Most communication and development projects are designed for funding periods of two to four years. In successful programs, that is usually enough time to achieve a reasonable degree of behavior change in a target audience. The opportunity to work on long-term maintenance of those behaviors is not as common, so the wealth of knowledge and field experience that health ministries and international organizations have accumulated in initiating new behaviors is not balanced with an equal wealth of experience in maintenance. Nonetheless, the behavioral concepts that follow can be applied in communication programs for maintenance, just as they were applied in the communication programs described earlier.

To present ideas in an understandable and logical order, we discuss maintenance separately from other behavioral and communication issues and have put the chapter near the end of the book. Yet, when one is actually planning and implementing communication projects, maintenance issues need to be addressed simultaneously with the assessment of the target audiences's practices and their consequences (for example, what positive consequences can the health and social system provide to maintain the target behavior?), the selection of target behaviors (which behaviors generate naturally occurring, recognizable consequences?), the selection of communication channels (which channels could convey messages most reliably over the long term?), and so on. Maintenance, then, is not one in a sequence of steps, but is an overlay of issues to be incorporated throughout the communication process.

Even though maintenance issues should be considered in the initial planning of communication programs, programs usually begin by emphasizing the introduction of new behaviors, and later the emphasis shifts to activities to maintain those behaviors. Because achieving maintenance is a long-term endeavor, however, programs focusing on behavior maintenance need a chance to produce data and feedback to planners and participants in order for the long-term effects of a particular approach to be evaluated.

Key Behavioral Principles

A discussion of maintaining health practices from a behavioral perspective and designing effective communication programs rests on three main ideas.

1. *To maintain behavior, events acting as prompts for the behavior (antecedents) still need to occur, the behavior itself needs to be performed correctly, and positive results need to follow (consequences).* In planning for maintenance, communicators need to assess target behaviors and, after those behaviors are learned, incorporate effective antecedents and consequences for supporting them.

2. *Most behaviors critical to carrying out child survival interventions are not inherently rewarding.* Many of them are preventive in nature and do not produce immediately apparent, positive results to encourage adoption as health practices. To survive as normal practices until their long-term (preventive) health benefits are recognized, these behaviors need support from the social network and health system.

3. *Conditions (antecedents and consequences) that effectively promote the trial or learning of new behaviors are not neces-*

sarily the optimal conditions for maintaining those behaviors over time (Sulzer-Azaroff & Mayer, 1977, pp. 428–429). In learning, target behaviors are broken down into steps; individuals are urged to practice these steps and are carefully given constructive and rewarding feedback. Programs introduce antecedents and consequences to support the learning process. Yet, once an individual is more or less fluent in the skill, many of these procedures and techniques are no longer necessary or feasible. Sometimes, naturally occurring antecedents and consequences will begin to support the behavior; so program supports might be reduced to occasional reminders or a community group providing social support.

Favorable conditions in the environment will help individuals maintain learned behaviors. The main objective of a maintenance program, then, is to put these conditions into place in order to create an environment of support for learned behaviors (Krasner, 1980). The major components of the program would be events in the environment that function as antecedents and consequences and are clearly linked to the behaviors targeted for maintenance. These "events in the environment" could be positive reactions from significant people, favorable policy changes, reminders over the radio, community groups advocating health practices, or health workers getting periodic, constructive feedback on their work.

Program Implications

The three behavioral concepts have the following implications for communication programs when they are shifting emphasis from initiation to maintenance of behavior.

- The communication methodology and behavioral principles discussed earlier still apply to maintenance, but different activities will be emphasized to focus more explicitly on supporting learned behavior, not introducing new behavior.
- Consequences introduced specifically to reinforce learning new behaviors should be faded out, and naturally occurring consequences from as many sources as possible should be strengthened (Miller, 1980, Chap. 18).
- Target audiences in maintenance programs are not just child

caretakers and mothers, but also include those people and organizations that can support mothers' and caretakers' health practices.

- The best choice for participation in successful maintenance programs are those individuals and organizations in the social and health systems who are already approximating supportive behaviors and actions for health practices.
- Any activity selected as part of a maintenance program must also generate its own positive consequences for participants, so that they will continue to support health practices without outside help.

The practice of exclusive breast feeding offers an example of a program emphasizing initiation or maintenance. The first several weeks of breast feeding for a first-time mother can be unrewarding at best, and many women abandon the practice prematurely. An effective communication program would offer training to the mother during prenatal visits or at the birthing site. Besides teaching breast-feeding skills, the program would provide strategies for overcoming potential breast-feeding problems. It would also provide social support (encouragement and constructive feedback), particularly in the early months of the new mother's experience. In contrast, a program for maintaining exclusive breast feeding for experienced mothers would not need to focus as intensely on the skills and benefits of breast feeding but would focus more on continued breast feeding when the mother returns to work and on instructions for introducing other foods and liquids and, later, weaning foods and practices. The naturally occurring positive consequences of breast feeding would be the critical ones maintaining the practice.

In summary, to design a program to maintain learned behaviors, communicators should go through the same steps of the communication methodology used to design behavior change initiation: *assess* the environment for current behaviors and activities that approximate support to desired health practices, *plan* the involvement of both the social and health care delivery systems in this supportive role, and then seek ways to *maintain* their involvement over the long term (Rasmuson, Seidel, Smith, & Booth, 1988). The ultimate purpose of these steps is to use communication to help design a supportive environment for the practice of child survival behaviors.

Assessing the Community and Health System for Sources of Support

When the communication goal is to maintain appropriate health practices in mothers and caretakers, one of the primary target audiences will be individuals who are key supporters of mothers' and caretakers' behaviors. Support for behavior, either engaging existing or creating new sources of support, is a critical part of a maintenance strategy. Many health practices promoted by communication programs are preventive in nature; do not produce immediately recognizable positive consequences; and are seen as ineffective, "a waste of time," or not worth the expense. So, to maintain preventive health practices over time, alternative sources of support need to be created or engaged until the long-term benefits of prevention become clear. For example, until the community as a whole sees that fewer of its children are dying during measles epidemics, health workers must reinforce parents for completing the immunization series.

Finding Sources of Support

Health practices are primarily influenced by two systems: one is the social system and community in which individuals live; the other is the formal and traditional health care delivery system. Figure 7.1 shows how a communicator might visualize the environment that supports health practices for children. The communicator's initial task in maintenance is to select as target audiences those people or organizations who can help individuals caring for the health of a young child.

Individuals are strongly influenced by the positive and negative reactions of people in their social network—close relatives, neighbors, and certain opinion leaders—to their health practices (McKinley, 1976). Therefore, communicators plan strategies to engage individuals in a mother's social network who could reinforce her efforts to practice child survival technologies. Communicators also look at what types of reinforcers could be used to influence the

Figure 7.1. Systems That Support Health Practices for Children.

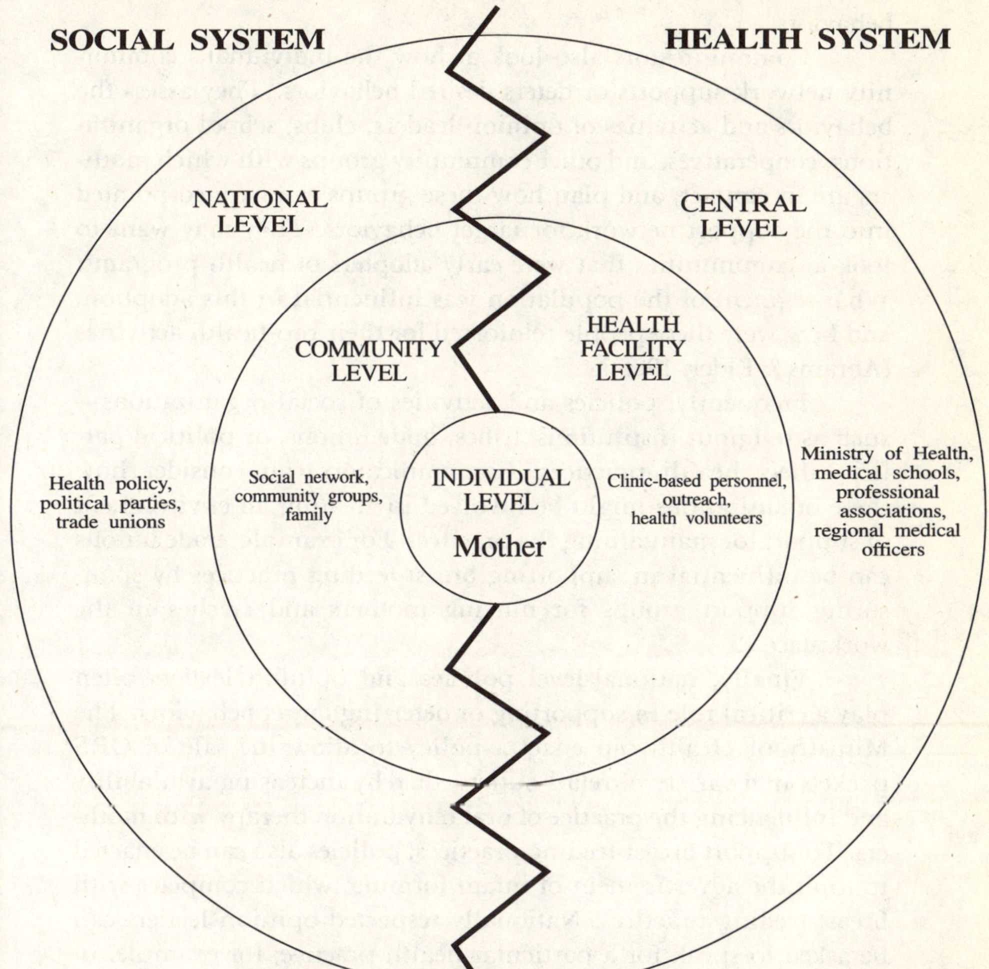

network's role in providing social support to the mother. Research can help the communicator discover which people are critical in supporting a mother and how they might be involved most effectively. In many societies, for example, a mother's female relatives are important in supporting child care practices. A woman's sisters, mother, and aunts could be mobilized or reinforced through a communication program to encourage or help in her practice of target behaviors.

Communicators also look at how the individual's community network supports or deters desired behaviors. They assess the behaviors and activities of opinion leaders, clubs, school organizations, cooperatives, and other community groups with which mothers are in contact, and plan how these groups can be incorporated into the support network for target behaviors. They may want to look at communities that were early adopters of health programs: What segment of the population was influential in this adoption, and how were these people reinforced for their pro-health activities (Abrams & Elder, 1986)?

Frequently, policies and activities of social organizations—such as religious institutions, tribes, trade unions, or political parties—affect health practices. Communicators can consider how these organizations might be involved in creating an environment of support for maintaining the practices. For example, trade unions can be influential in supporting breast-feeding practices by sponsoring support groups for nursing mothers and crèches in the workplace.

Finally, national-level policies and opinion leaders often play a critical role in supporting or deterring target behaviors. The Ministry of Health can enact a policy to allow the sale of ORS packets in a variety of retail outlets, thereby increasing availability and influencing the practice of oral rehydration therapy with mothers. To support breast-feeding practices, policies also can be enacted to limit the advertisement of infant formula, which competes with breast-feeding practices. Nationally respected opinion leaders can be asked to speak for a particular health practice; for example, in television spots during a measles immunization campaign in the Philippines, opinion leaders such as the minister of health and a leading television personality promoted the program (Verzosa, Bernaje, de Guzman, Hernandez, Reodica, & Taguiwalo, 1989).

Communicators should also look for support from the various levels of the formal health care delivery system. As shown in Figure 7.1, the health system is made up of a variety of professionals: village-based health workers, clinic-based nurses and doctors, their immediate supervisors, regional inspectors, and central-level Ministry of Health staff. A communication strategy needs to be devised to help these professionals and volunteers support mothers' behavior. Communication strategies can work as antecedents to change policy, improve supply and clinic procedures, or improve the supervisory skills of communication supervisors. Communication strategies can also work as consequences to improve patient-client interaction, strengthen outreach activities, and give recognition to program successes.

In many countries, traditional healers and birth attendants are active and influential in the health domain. They often have close ties with the community and can reach mothers who are not in contact with the formal medical system. Sometimes traditional healers are organized into associations and can be approached collectively; sometimes they need to be approached individually. Nevertheless, they often can be useful in communicating with mothers and supporting their health practices.

A critical component to the long-term success of a communication program is maintaining effective practices of workers at all levels of the health care delivery system. Their role as the "front-line" interpersonal contact with mothers is essential in maintaining health practices. Health workers are asked to learn and practice many skills in order to teach and support mothers' health practices. A communication program needs to consider the conditions in which health workers themselves work, and to apply behavioral principles to assess and improve the environment to maintain their behaviors. Only when these health workers are supported in the practice of learned communication and case management skills can they be counted on as reliable sources of reinforcement and support to mothers (Reis, Elder, Satoto, Kodyat, & Palmer, 1990; Elder et al., 1992).

Finding Approximations, Antecedents, and Consequences

Communicators should search the social and health systems for what is already working to some extent (approximations) and determine why it is working (what antecedents and consequences support those activities). Currently active organizations and people signal to communicators that positive consequences for their functions already exist, so these organizations and people are good candidates for participation in a maintenance program. Rather than having to create something new (will the new system be viable over the long term?), communicators can provide existing organizations and individuals with materials and planned activities specific to supporting mothers' child survival practices. For example, in urban areas, trade unions or factories may already have viable programs that address the health and family needs of workers. These unions and employers may have found that such programs attract more union members or lower employee turnover (positive consequence to sustain the factory's or trade union's support of the employees). The network among local market women may be another communication channel to tap. Over the years, exchanging useful information or helping each other has paid off in a variety of ways (positive outcomes that maintain the network). If grandmothers play an influential role in child rearing, they might also be engaged in the maintenance system. Fulfilling their role as good grandmothers is an esteemed function in the community (which is a social consequence maintaining their behavior).

The same principles apply when one is assessing the health care delivery side of the circle in Figure 7.1 for approximations to effective maintenance activities. In other words, communicators can look for existing activities and structures that could play a role in supporting child survival interventions. Individual health workers might already be conducting outreach to remind mothers who are behind in the immunization schedule (approximation). They find the mothers more receptive and interactive when approached at home and enjoy getting out of the clinic periodically (naturally occurring consequences). A regional hospital has opened an oral rehydration unit (approximation) and, as a result, receives visits from Ministry of Health officials and donors to observe an oral rehydration unit in action (positive, observable consequence). Traditional birth attendants deliver most of the babies in rural areas (approximation). Mothers openly recognize them as health experts (positive, observable consequence). These activities, although not yet specifically supporting behaviors targeted for mothers, naturally result in positive consequences and so could be considered as viable, long-term communication channels.

Differentiating Between Skill and Performance Deficits

The assessment process will reveal not only what is working in both the social and health care delivery systems but also what is not working. Individual skills and knowledge often are fairly high, and the most likely obstacles to long-term maintenance of target behaviors fall in the category of performance deficits. In other words, adequate support for desired behavior is lacking. A woman may be so overburdened with child-rearing, farming, marketing, and home maintenance responsibilities that, despite knowledge of and belief in the value of immunizations, she cannot respect the schedule with her present infant. A health worker may have been trained in effective health communication techniques, but the case load as it is presently handled at the clinic does not allow him to exchange information with mothers. A regional medical inspector likes the idea of checklists to monitor case management and communication skills of the staff of oral rehydration units in local health centers, but most of his time is spent preparing reports for the central office, and maintaining a private practice to support the family. Visiting the units and initiating a monitoring scheme have become low priority. Moreover, since the Ministry of Health has not mandated a monitoring system, the additional effort to put such a system in place would go unrecognized. These examples illustrate how skills and performance deficits might affect the maintenance of desired practices in the health system.

Planning Communication Strategies for Maintenance

In planning for maintenance, it is important to engage the interdisciplinary team that helped plan the initial communication program. The composition of the team would necessarily change to include administrators, community leaders, and representatives of organizations that will play a role in maintenance. In attempting to plan long-term support for appropriate health practices in a target audience, the team cannot repair every weakness in the health care delivery or social system. Because of the limited amount of resources and time usually allotted to putting effective programs in place, focusing on maintenance strategies in some order of priority is essential in the planning process. With these priorities clearly in mind, the team should, as before, review and select target behaviors, develop communication strategies, and select communication channels specifically to maintain health practices. In selecting target behaviors, the team should consider two types of behaviors. First are the mothers' health practices: breast feeding, hand washing, getting prenatal care and immunizations, giving fluids and food during diarrhea, and taking children with pneumonia symptoms to a health care facility. Second are behaviors that support health practices: health workers' communication and case management skills, fathers providing money for transportation to the clinic, volunteers distributing ORS packets and mixing information, and community groups offering help to breast-feeding women. The interdisciplinary team should decide which target behaviors will have the most impact on maintaining the changes already accomplished.

In general, communication strategies for maintenance will do one or several of the following:

- Fade out any consequences created to introduce new behaviors.
- Strengthen existing positive consequences for the behavior.
- Eliminate or change any negative consequences.
- Use antecedents to remind individuals of important information (time, place, availability).

As much as possible, the team should incorporate these components into an existing activity that reaches the target audience and is already generating positive consequences for the participants.

Communication channels play a role both as antecedents and as consequences to behavior maintenance. Interpersonal communication, radio and television spots, print materials, and newspaper ads can all remind, review important information, and reward. Communicators, then, need to decide which function will best maintain target behaviors and which channel can best fulfill that function over the long term. The personal congratulations from a health worker may be more effective in helping a mother finish the immunization series than a poster on the clinic wall saying "Good Mothers Immunize Their Children." But what can be done to ensure that the health worker continues to congratulate mothers over the years? In choosing this channel over others, communicators would have to take into consideration the cost of maintaining health workers as a communication channel. In other cases, if coverage rates are already fairly high in a region, periodic radio reminders to come to the clinic for immunizations may be enough to maintain the rate.

Other Maintenance-Related Communication Issues

Generally, maintenance activities should focus on generating positive consequences for health practices. Recognition and constructive feedback are two nonmaterial rewards that can do much to maintain health practices. A communication activity might be to teach health workers how to give mothers feedback on their weaning practices or their skill in administering ORS to a child that vomits. If the health workers' behavior is considered critical to maintaining mothers' health practices, then effective supervision, through recognition and constructive feedback to health workers, might be the major activity for a maintenance program. Further training, for example, could shift from simple instruction to problem solving. Health workers themselves could set the training agenda to address problems encountered when using communication techniques with mothers. Supervisors can give recognition by using solutions provided by the group. Chapter Five gives more suggestions on how training can be used as a positive consequence for health workers.

Communication activities focusing on maintenance of health behaviors can be monitored in the same way as activities serving mostly to teach and motivate new behaviors. As discussed in Chapter Six, monitoring itself can be used as a key strategy in maintaining people's behaviors in both the social and health care delivery systems. If properly functioning, monitoring will generate vital information on how well systems are supporting desired health practices. It can then be shown to participants, donors, and other decision makers as feedback, reinforcement, and the basis for deciding future directions.

Maintaining Initial Gains: The Honduran Example

A communication program that has been funded for over ten years in Honduras allows us to examine the program's effectiveness in maintaining initial gains made in health practices.

A communication pilot project was implemented in Honduras from 1981 to 1983, for the purpose of establishing widespread use of oral rehydration therapy (ORT) in the home to combat dehydration and diarrhea among children under five years of age. While the central feature of ORT is the administration of an oral rehydration solution (ORS), the therapy also encompasses nutritional and feeding behaviors, such as continued breast feeding and other feeding and increased liquid intake. In Honduras, the rehydration solution is called Litrosol, which is mixed from locally produced packets containing the ORS powdered formula.

In 1982, after the pilot project had proved successful in one health region, the Ministry of Health began a diarrheal disease control program to serve all areas of the country. The national effort, involving continued technical assistance from the Academy for Educational Development and funding from the United States Agency for International Development, remains active to the present. National ORT promotion is based on the communication methodology developed during the pilot project, integrating broadcast and print media with interpersonal communication to reach its audience. Under the national program, the intensive use of radio necessary for the learning phase of the program was reduced, and more emphasis was placed on promoting ORT via health workers. A follow-up evaluation survey was conducted in 1987 to determine whether behavior changes occurring in 1983 had been sustained.

One target behavior from this project illustrates issues affecting its maintenance since the initiation of the communication program: mothers' responses to the question "Have you treated the most recent case (past two weeks) of diarrhea with Litrosol?" From a baseline taken in 1981 of 9.2 percent of the cases being treated with Litrosol, the two-year campaign resulted in mothers reporting that

35.7 percent were being treated with Litrosol (1983). The follow-up survey showed a continued trend toward adoption (44.8 percent).

What Events Are Supporting Honduran Mothers' Use of ORT?

What events are currently operating to support mothers' continued use of ORT? Are these events functioning as antecedents or consequences? Are they coming from program activities, the social environment, or the health care delivery system? Are they coming from the practice itself? Answers to these questions will help program planners design program messages and activities specifically to support and maintain mothers' behavior.

Messages. The messages from all channels have positioned Litrosol as a treatment for dehydration, not for diarrhea. This is an antecedent strategy that helps increase the positive impact of the following consequence: using the product made signs of dehydration disappear or kept the child from displaying the signs during the bout of diarrhea. Indeed, mothers' reported belief that Litrosol stopped diarrhea fell from 58 percent in 1983 to 22 percent in 1987. Conversely, their belief that it avoided dehydration rose from 20 percent to 59 percent. The evaluation data demonstrate that this knowledge was converted into an antecedent for the desired behavior; as case severity increased, so did mothers' use of Litrosol. ORS was administered in 40 percent of cases that mothers judged as mild, in 46 percent of cases judged as moderate, and in 54 percent of cases considered severe.

Health Care Delivery System. The research shows that mothers who were in contact with the health care delivery system were more likely to use Litrosol to treat the most recent case than mothers who were out of contact. Over five hundred health care workers were trained in communication skills, and it is likely that through their efforts they are reinforcing mothers either through providing praise, encouragement, and discussion or being a credible source of information. In some way, they are giving positive attention to mothers engaging in this behavior.

The Media Mix. For various reasons, radio was not used as intensely during the national ORT promotion as during the pilot project. The data indicate that the use of radio, systematically integrated with print and interpersonal communication, helped to create an environment of support for the maintenance of ORT use. Evaluation data are consistently higher on all measures—from trial use to case treatment rates—for the pilot project area than for the national program. The evaluators concluded that since the pilot project relied heavily on mass communication to support ORT information transmitted by health workers and the current strategy relies principally on health workers and small-scale alternative media, the original mix of communication channels was probably more effective than the current emphasis on interpersonal channels.

The Behavior Itself. Clearly, the use of some form of ORT is *not* competing with other treatments, rather, mothers seem to use it in conjunction with other remedies. On the positive side, their use of breast feeding and home-available fluids, which was fairly high in 1983, has remained high even with increased use of Litrosol. The negative practice of purging has gone down, from 50 percent in 1983 to 24 percent in 1987. Unfortunately, their use of antidiarrheals has gone up, from 25 percent to 64 percent over the same time period. Seventy percent provided more than one treatment to their child during the diarrhea episode, indicating that ORT did not replace competing behaviors but, rather, was added on to what mothers were already doing.

To improve the maintenance system for proper treatment of diarrhea and dehydration, the program may want to weaken the support for prescribing and administering medicine, since increasing the use of ORS alone has not replaced this practice. According to mothers, health centers recommended medicine as a treatment more often than ORS (69 percent medicine and 57 percent ORS), whereas community-based health workers recommended ORS more often (22 percent medicine, 78 percent ORS, and 37 percent going to a health center). (Note that more than one treatment could be recommended (Baume, 1988)). Clinic-based health workers, nurses, and doctors then may become new target audiences for building a maintenance system for mothers' behavior. Program interventions can reach them at their work or through their professional associations and medical and nursing schools. Private or parastatal pharmaceutical companies might also be brought on as supportive partners for ORS use if meaningful incentives were clearly available.

What Can We Learn About Maintenance from Honduras?

Although this example has not provided clear-cut answers to how to maintain behavior change, it has generated questions that public health and communication professionals will be considering in conceptualizing future programs.

Communication Issues

- What is the effect of the initial program intensity on planning and development and communication?
- What indirect benefits from the communication program can be identified (for example, the health system's preparedness for the emergence of cholera or overall attitudes in the population toward the health system)?
- What conclusions can we draw about the levels of intensity of communication programs necessary to sustain public awareness? Are reminders all that are necessary?
- How can communication programs geared for maintaining health practices accommodate women newly entering motherhood?
- Can long-term effects of mortality be detected?

Broader Programmatic Issues

- Has the Ministry of Health adopted a sound health communication methodology?
- Have communication skills been incorporated into health care professionals' training?
- Is the target behavior embedded within the social context of the population?
- Are private sector and other organizations demonstrating good program-planning and implementation skills?

- What are the optimal necessary levels of financial and logistical support to nurture the project (what level of support was necessary to sustain the ministry's correct use the communication methodology?) and to wean the project (how can program support disengage without losing the benefits of the investment?)?

Summary

In the past two decades, we have learned much about the impact that communication can have on health behavior but we still have much to learn about the maintenance of behavior change. Health communicators have been typically asked to create programs to produce impressive behavior changes. But when donors and policy makers move on to other priorities, and the years go by, what is there to show for those initial expensive and labor-intensive efforts? Is the system put into place having any long-term effect on saving children from illness and death? Or have most of the behavior change gains eroded over time because of a lack of focused social and logistical support? These are the issues that now need the same careful planning, monitoring, creativity, and innovation invested in earlier communication programs. Specifically:

- Maintenance programs should be explicitly planned, funded, and implemented.
- The communication methodology and behavioral principles discussed earlier still apply to maintenance, but different activities will be emphasized to focus more explicitly on supporting learned behavior rather than on introducing new behavior.
- Consequences introduced specifically to reinforce the learning of new behaviors should be faded out, and naturally occurring consequences from as many sources as possible should be strengthened.
- Target audiences in maintenance programs are not just the children's caretakers and mothers but also the people and organizations that can support mothers' and caretakers' health practices.
- The best choices for participation in successful maintenance programs are those individuals and organizations in the social

and health systems who are already approximating supportive behaviors and actions for health practices.

- Any activity selected as part of a maintenance program must also generate its own positive consequences for participants, so that they will continue to support health practices without outside help.

By continuing to focus on observable behavior—even when considering organization and community involvement—program managers can apply many principles and tools used earlier to initiate behavior change to maintain these changes over time. While the ultimate goal is to maintain *individual* health practices, in applying behavioral principles, program managers can incorporate broader social and health systems to support those practices over the long term.

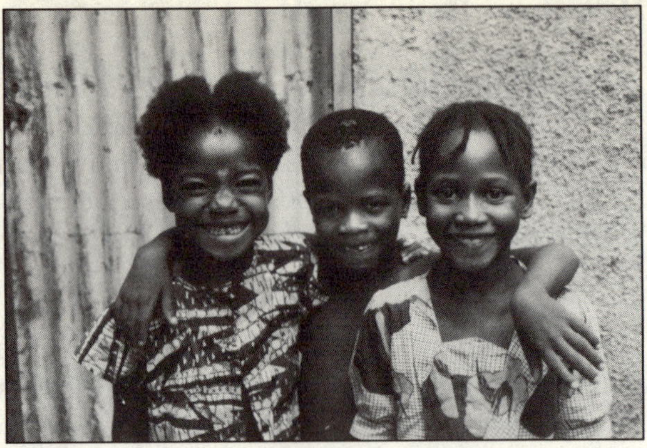

8

Lessons and Implications for Future Work

Writing this book has given us an opportunity to reflect on the last fifteen years of our communication experience. As we gathered and reviewed materials from the various projects in a multitude of countries, we also talked informally with public health professionals both here and abroad about their experience with behavior change. This what they had to say:

"Some people have very strong misconceptions or stereotypes about behavior analysis and the vocabulary we use to talk about it." Some people would stop listening when we mentioned the words *consequences* or *antecedents.* We found that the people who ignored the "historical baggage" that behavior analysis carries or who were not tied to any one theory of communication or behavior were more open to applying the principles and techniques coming from behavior analysis.

"This behavioral approach is user friendly." It was interesting to see how a variety of health professionals in our country—physicians, health program managers, communication specialists, health educators, trainers, nurses, and community volunteers—

could apply the behavioral approach in their work. Once they understood the basic principles, they could design their own strategy, instruments, and tools specifically for their own communication activities.

"This behavioral approach travels well because it accommodates differences among cultures." Because behavior analysis focuses on observable behavior and the observable events in the environment that influence it, we could look directly at how the behavior functioned within our own culture. We knew to look for events triggering a behavior and events supporting or weakening it; yet the form that those events would take differed from one culture to another. Even within our own country, communication strategies were different, depending on the cultural context of a target audience.

"Catch them doing something right!" The principle of rewarding and shaping behavioral approximations made a big difference in the way we approached communication and training. We had been mostly focusing on programmatic constraints and what people were doing poorly or incorrectly, and we were not building on what programs and people were doing well. This new, more positive strategy made people more willing to try suggestions for improvement.

"I didn't have to do it all at once." One of the principles of behavior analysis is to break actions down into measurable steps and to shape behavior by rewarding those steps. We found that we could apply this approach to our own use of behavior analysis. We started with applying it to one piece of our communication work. We tried using direct observation as a research technique; trainers tried giving homework during their training session and following up later; or sometimes we tried applying the Behavior Analysis Scale (Resource E) to help us select and put target behaviors in order of priority. We found that we did not have to tackle everything all at once but, rather, could try the approach in one step of the communication process, learn from that experience, and go on from there.

"Behaviors aren't what you think they are." Behaviors are much more complex than we originally thought. Behavior analysis provided tools to help us actually observe those behaviors and understand their complexity and the events that preceded and followed them. It helped put a microscope on behavior, which made us understand that what we originally thought was one action was actually a series of steps. We used those steps to design skill-based training and develop more specific messages for our communication program.

"Every behavior is constantly getting beaten up by other behaviors." There is a lot of competition out there. Many health behaviors especially preventive behaviors that do not seem to lead to any recognizable outcomes—need support from time to time to stay high on people's priority lists. We cannot just teach people once, or even twice. We need to plan reminders, refreshers, rewards, and recognition into our communication programs, to be sure that important preventive health practices do not get lost.

"It takes more than improved health behaviors to improve health." As time went on, we saw that behavior change was necessary in more than just mothers' health practices; and we were pleased to see that behavioral principles could apply to *all* behavior, not just health behaviors. For example, for any behavior needed to run our program—whether monitoring or training or supervising—we still needed to consider how antecedents and consequences would affect the performance of those behaviors too.

"The concept that we needed to consider the consequences was the 'big idea' for me." We knew that knowledge was not enough to lead to behavior change, but we found that teaching and shaping skills were not enough either. In many cases, people knew what they should do and they knew *how;* yet they still weren't doing an effective job. If we looked closely, we saw that people often got punishment or no reaction at all for their actions. What we needed to do was consider how consequences supported or weakened health practices as we developed our communication strategies. Using this behavioral approach helped us find strategies that took consequences

into account and supported people in applying their knowledge and skills. Our search for sources of positive consequences to support people in their efforts led us to their social and professional networks and the community at large.

Looking Forward

What about the future? What will be some of the future applications and directions for applying behavior analysis to change and support healthy practices? Once again, the discussions with people who have been applying these principles and techniques provided some ideas.

"We've learned a lot how to introduce new behaviors and skills related to child survival, but we haven't had a chance yet to apply behavioral principles to the maintenance of those behaviors." The funding for many of the communication programs described in this book ended just when the levels of behavior change had reached the level necessary to apply the principles described in the chapter on maintenance. In the future, we need to plan our health programs in such a way as to provide time and funding for health communication to focus explicitly on behavior maintenance.

"Couldn't we use the same behavioral principles and techniques and apply them to strengthening the capacity of the Ministry of Health and other institutions to engage in effective health communication?" Communicators could follow the same principles for individual behavior change, yet adapt and apply them to institutional change:

- Define objectives for institutional capacity building in terms of *observable actions to be taken.*
- Observe the institution's current actions related to these objectives. Analyze the actions for their relationship to the political, social, cultural, and physical environments in which they operate—the antecedents and consequences that help determine whether institutional actions will be repeated. Perform the same analysis for any institutional actions that compete with health communication methodology.
- Design and implement a strategy that will increase the desired

institutional actions and at the same time create an environment of support for them. In some institutions, we might have to focus first on developing skills of key personnel. In others, where the skills necessary for conducting health communication already exist, the strategy might focus on increasing positive consequences or reducing negative consequences by changing policy, establishing norms, and creating rewards.

- Measure observable indicators of the target actions. Follow these indicators before and during communication program activities.
- Use the results of this measurement as constructive feedback to institutional members to strengthen the desired actions.

"We need to take the human factor more into account as we develop new, and adapt existing, child survival technologies." The link between technology and health is people's behavior; we need to incorporate that link when we are developing those technologies. Too frequently, technologies and procedures are developed in laboratories and hospitals, and no thought is given to the people who will use these technologies in their daily lives. Many child survival technologies are not intrinsically rewarding and in some cases are actually punishing to do. Immunizations can induce fever in a well child. ORS does not stop diarrhea, and it can cause a child to vomit if it is administered too rapidly. The growth-monitoring chart is a complex visual aid that many mothers do not understand; therefore, it does not provide the reinforcement that it was originally designed to provide. Vitamin A capsules seem to have no effect whatsoever on a child. Increased hand washing can actually punish the mother, who must carry the extra water it requires great distances to her home. As new technologies are developed and health professionals attempt to adapt them to their programs, they need to consider the consequences and the complexity of behavior these technologies require. The continued use of child survival technologies will greatly increase if they are more intrinsically rewarding and feasible and if they provide immediate, salient consequences to the child and the caretakers.

"We really are becoming a global community and the health problems we face are becoming more similar." This statement has

several implications for the application of behavior analysis to introduce and support health practices in both developing and industrialized countries. (1) The priority health problems are changing. As infant mortality is being reduced, many developing countries, such as Indonesia, Brazil, and Costa Rica, are facing issues related to chronic disease and life-style practices. At the same time, many industrialized countries are seeing an increase in infant mortality from diarrhea and the resurgence of immunizable diseases. What we have learned about applying behavior analysis to child survival in developing countries could also be valuable to industrialized countries. (2) The world is becoming more diverse. Population growth and migration patterns between countries are making industrialized countries more heterogeneous every day. Experience in infectious disease control and child survival, work with large populations with limited resources, and efforts to meet the special needs of these populations (cultural, linguistic, and socioeconomic)—all have increasing relevance to public health programs in the United States and other industrialized countries. (3) Resources, even in industrialized countries, are becoming scarcer. Health professionals around the world are working to make health care more cost-efficient and effective. Increasingly, we are learning that preventing illness is less expensive than treating it, and that one of the keys to prevention is behavior change on a large scale. Throughout the upcoming decade, we will need to do much more to help people change their own behaviors in order to lead longer and healthier lives. To assist them as they work toward that goal, behavior analysis offers health professionals an approach that is simple, straightforward, and easily measurable. (4) Environmental issues related to the air, water, and soil will need immediate and coordinated action. In order to save our planet, governments, businesses, communities, and individuals will need to change their behaviors in ways and at levels never before considered.

Health professionals at Alma-Ata called for "Health for All by the Year 2000." There is still a great deal to be done. Indeed, there is still a great deal to be learned about the role that communication and behavior change can take, as we work together to support a healthier community, country, and planet.

Resource: The Communicator's Toolbox for Behavior Change

The following checklists can help communicators focus more explicitly on behavior change at each step of the communication process: assessment, planning, training, and monitoring. Each checklist, however, should be adapted to reflect the characteristics of the selected behavior and the cultural and demographic factors of the country in which the instrument is to be used. The adapted checklists should be tested and revised before they are applied.

A. Performance Observation Checklist: Health Worker's Counseling Skills with Individual Mothers. This checklist could be used by trainers, supervisors, or the health workers themselves to assess interpersonal counseling skills during health worker–client interaction. The first section (a generic checklist) can be adapted to any technical health issue. The second (an observation checklist) is used specifically for immunization counseling skills.

B. Performance Observation Checklist: Health Worker's Group Presentation Interpersonal Skills. This checklist could be used by trainers, supervisors, or the health workers themselves to assess group presentation skills during a health talk.

C. Ideal Behavior and Observation Checklist: Breast Feeding. The Ideal Behavior lists the target behaviors for correct breast feeding. The observation checklist could be used during a two- to four-hour observation period by communicators to help shape or monitor the communication strategy. It could also be used by a lactation counselor to assess to what degree the breast-feeding skills she is promoting are being adopted.

D. Performance Observation Checklist: Hand Washing. This checklist could be used as a part of an in-depth interview or survey to observe hand-washing behaviors promoted as a part of a diarrheal disease prevention program. It could be applied during assessment or during a health promoter's home visit or to monitor behavior change.

E. Selecting Target Behaviors: The Behavior Analysis Scale. This scale could be used by the interdisciplinary planning team to organize discussions related to the selection of target behaviors after assessment has been conducted.

F. Selecting Target Behaviors: Target Behavior Selection Worksheets. These worksheets also can assist an interdisciplinary planning team in selecting target behaviors after assessment has been conducted.

G. Planning for Behavior Change Checklist. This checklist could be used to assist communicators in planning a communication program that focuses explicitly on behavior change and maintenance.

H. Training for Behavior Change Checklist. This checklist could be used by trainers to assist in the design and implementation of skills-based training.

I. Monitoring for Behavior Change Checklist. This checklist could be used by communicators, trainers, supervisors, and clinic staff to monitor behavior change and use the monitoring data as feedback to maintain target behaviors. The first section could be adapted by anyone interested in monitoring behavior change; the second could be used by a supervisor monitoring interpersonal communication skills at the clinic level.

A. PERFORMANCE OBSERVATION CHECKLIST: HEALTH WORKER'S COUNSELING SKILLS WITH INDIVIDUAL MOTHERS

Generic Checklist

____ Greets mother.
____ Smiles at mother.
____ Asks open-ended question about mother's experience.
____ Praises specific action(s) that mother has done correctly.
____ Advises mother about specific actions she should do next.
____ Asks mother to explain what she has just heard.
____ Praises mother for what she has repeated correctly.
____ Corrects specific messages that mother has not repeated.
____ Asks mother what problems or constraints she might have in carrying out what health worker is recommending.
____ Discusses with the mother what she can do to resolve the problem or constraint.
____ Uses appropriate vocabulary (the specific words selected would be based on the cultural and linguistic setting).
____ Asks mother if she has any questions concerning what she has heard or anything about the health of her child.
____ Praises/thanks mother for coming.

Individual Counseling Skills Applied to Immunizations

____ Greets mother.
____ Smiles at mother.
____ Praises mother for having brought her child to the health center to be immunized.
____ Asks mother if she has any questions about the immunizations or other aspects of her child's health.
____ Explains what side effects might occur from this immunization (if appropriate).
____ Explains what to do in case of side effects.
____ Asks mother what she will do if her baby gets sick tonight.
____ Praises mother for what she has repeated correctly.

____ Corrects specific information concerning side effects which the mother has not repeated.

____ Asks mother what problems or constraints she might have in carrying out this recommendation.

____ Discusses with the mother what she can do to resolve the problem or constraint.

____ Explains how many vaccinations the child needs to complete his or her immunization schedule.

____ Explains date and time mother should return.

____ Asks mother how many vaccinations the child needs to complete immunization schedule and specifies the date and time mother should return.

____ Asks mother what problems she might have in returning to complete the immunizations.

____ Praises/reinforces mother for what she has repeated correctly.

____ Corrects specific information concerning the number of vaccinations, and date and time mother should return, that the mother has not repeated.

____ Asks mother what problems or constraints she might have in bringing her child for immunizations at this time and date.

____ Discusses with the mother what she can do to resolve the problem or constraint.

____ Uses appropriate vocabulary. (Specific words would be based on the health topic and the cultural and linguistic setting.)

____ Asks mother if she has any other questions.

____ If so, repeats the question mother has asked.

____ Explains answer.

____ Asks mother what she has heard.

____ Thanks mother again for coming.

____ Repeats that she will see her again at the specific time and date the mother should return.

B. PERFORMANCE OBSERVATION CHECKLIST: HEALTH WORKER'S GROUP PRESENTATION SKILLS

Check the frequency of the following health worker actions:

Skills	Frequency
Asks open-ended questions.	
Asks closed-ended questions.	
Uses appropriate language (specific words selected would be based on the health topic and the cultural and linguistic setting).	
Asks mothers if they have any questions.	
Restates mother's question before answering it.	
Asks mothers to respond to questions as a group.	

Check off if the health worker does the following:

____ 1. Greets mothers individually.

____ 2. States health topic.

____ 3. States purpose of session.

____ 4. Asks at least one mother to share experiences concerning the topic.

____ 5. Restates mothers' comments or experiences.

____ 6. Congratulates mother(s) for a good health practice or healthy baby.

____ 7. Demonstrates target behaviors (mixing ORS, for example).

____ 8. Has a mother or mothers demonstrate the target behaviors.

____ 14. Asks women to applaud (or praise in a culturally appropriate way) the mother(s) demonstrating the target behaviors.

____ 15. Tells mother(s) specifically what actions were done correctly in the demonstration.

____ 16. Tells mothers specifically what actions can be improved next time.

____ 17. Summarizes vital information covered during the session.

____ 18. Asks mothers to do something related to the target behaviors as soon as they get home.

____ 19. Asks mothers to share what they have learned with their husbands, other wives, and/or mothers-in-law when they get home.

____ 20. Asks mothers to sing a song.

____ 21. Involves mothers in a sociodrama or skit.

____ 22. Uses a fable/story/metaphor (for example, dried-out plant to explain dehydration) during the presentation.

Checklist of Teaching Aids

Check off if the health worker uses the following:

____ Brochure/leaflet/flyer distributed to mothers to take home

____ Flip chart

____ Poster

____ Flannelgram

____ Samples (ORS packets, syringes, etc.)

____ Blackboard

____ Other ______________________________

C. IDEAL BEHAVIOR AND OBSERVATION CHECKLIST: BREAST FEEDING

Note: Breast feeding is not a "technology" developed in a laboratory or university. It has been described as "the choreography of the dance between the mother and the baby." In contrast to its role in other child survival technologies, such as immunizations and growth monitoring, the infant is a major actor in breast feeding and greatly influences the practice. Because the practice is an interaction between the infant and the mother, it was more difficult to develop a "performance checklist" that would cut across all breast-feeding situations. The following checklist describes behaviors that contribute to the "choreography" of breast feeding. It includes some behaviors that are not absolutely necessary for "correct breast feeding" but are important indicators of the interaction between the mother and the child. This checklist should be reviewed locally and specific behaviors selected by an interdisciplinary team. As with all checklists, it should be tested before being applied on a wider scale.

This checklist was developed in coordination with Rukhsana Haider, International Center for Diarrhoeal Disease Control (International Center for Diarrheal Disease Research, Bangladesh), Dhaka, Bangladesh, and reviewed by Elena Hurtado (Nutrition Institute of Central America and Panama), Chloe O'Gara and Judy Canahuati (WELLSTART International), and Dr. F. Savage King (Programme for Control of Diarrheal Diseases, World Health Organization). The behaviors that seem to be the most critical to breast feeding have been starred.

ATTACHMENT TO THE BREAST

____ *1. Infant's mouth opens wide when it is put to the breast.

____ *2. Infant's lower lip is turned out when it is put to the breast.

____ 3. Mother brings baby to breast, not the breast to the baby.

____ *4. Infant's mouth covers a portion of areola, not just the nipple.

____ *5. Infant's mouth takes in more of the bottom tissues of the areola than the top tissue.

____ *6. Infant's chin is against the mother's breast.

____ *7. Infant's sucking is visibly rhymic and coordinated. (In the first few minutes, there are shallower, more rapid sucks. The rate after the first few minutes decreases—slower, deeper sucks—and then increases again.)

POSITION

____ *1. Infant's face is turned toward mother's breast. (Infants under two months old.)
____ 2. Infant's neck is straight (not twisted to one side).
____ 3. Infant's body is in a straight line (not twisted).
____ 4. Newborn's bottom is supported (if mother is sitting).

SEPARATION FROM THE BREAST

____ *1. Infant is relaxed/happy at the end of feeding, OR
____ Infant falls asleep while breast feeding.

If infant is awake after breast feeding:

____ 2. Infant comes off breast by himself to end the feeding session.
____ 3. Infant releases the breast easily.
____ 4. Infant does not cry after feeding session.
____ 5. If infant cries, mother returns infant to the breast.

If infant falls asleep while breast feeding:

____ 6. Mother uses finger to release the infant's mouth from the breast.

UNRESTRICTED FEEDING

____ 1. Mother breast-feeds when infant cries.
____ *2. Mother breast-feeds when infant shows visible hunger (rooting, for example).
____ *3. Mother breast-feeds when infant shows visible comfort-seeking behavior.

FEEDING AT NIGHT

____ *1. Infant sleeps with mother.
____ *2. Infant sleeps in same room, close to mother.

BONDING WITH THE MOTHER

(NOTE: These behaviors are not essential for successful breast feeding but are indicators of healthy attachment.)

____ 1. Mother smiles at infant while infant is feeding.
____ 2. Mother talks to/sings to infant while infant is feeding.
____ 3. Mother looks infant in the eyes while infant is feeding.
____ 4. Mother hugs/touches infant when infant is not feeding.
____ 5. Mother looks at infant when infant is not feeding.
____ 6. Mother talks to/sings to infant while infant is not feeding.

No. of Feeds	*Duration	Breast Utilized	
		Left	**Right**
Feed 1			
Feed 2			
Feed 3			
Feed 4			
Feed 5			

D. PERFORMANCE OBSERVATION CHECKLIST: HAND WASHING

MATERIALS NECESSARY FOR HAND WASHING

Material	**At Hand**	**Had to Look for It**
____ 1. Soap		
____ 2. Water that has not been used for another purpose		
____ 3. Clean towel or cloth		

HAND-WASHING STEPS

____ 1. Uses water that has not been used for any other purpose.
____ 2. Wets hands with running water.
____ 3. Soaps the hands.
____ 4. Rubs hands together until there is foam.
____ 5. Runs water over the hands until the soap is removed.
____ 6. If necessary, repeats the previous five steps until all dirt is removed.
7. Dries hands without recontaminating them by:
   a. Waving them in the air
   b. Drying them on a clean towel/cloth
   c. Other
____ 8. Washes hands before feeding child under three years old.
____ 9. Washes hands before preparing food.

DURATION OF EACH HAND WASHING

HAND WASHING	DURATION
#1	
#2	
#3	
#4	

Note: Some countries are promoting the use of ash rather than soap.

Source: Courtesy of Elena Hurtado, Nutrition Institute of Central America and Panama.

E. SELECTING TARGET BEHAVIORS: THE BEHAVIOR ANALYSIS SCALE

The Behavior Analysis Scale is a tool communicators can use during planning to select target behaviors. The scale includes nine aspects of behavior against which a potential target behavior can be rated from 0 to 5. Its resulting "score" helps planners see which of many behaviors are most amenable to change and which have the most potential for impact on the health problem.

The Behavior Analysis Scale helps to guide the interdisciplinary team in comparing formative research findings with the detailed list of discrete, behavioral steps necessary to perform the health practice. Applying the scale gives each potential target behavior a score acccording to how it fits in with nine dimensions considered crucial in producing behavior change. The higher its score, the more likely the behavior could be affected by a communication program.

STEPS IN APPLYING THE BEHAVIOR ANALYSIS SCALE

STEP 1: **Identify the ideal, medically prescribed behavioral steps in the sequential order** that the target audience would take in order to prevent or treat the health problem.

STEP 2: **Rate potential target behaviors.** The Behavior Analysis Scale breaks potential target behaviors down into nine categories:

- **What impact** do potential target behaviors have on the health problem being addressed?
- **Do they have positive consequences** that are immediately perceivable to the person performing the behavior?
- **Are they compatible** with what the person is already doing? The behavior may not presently exist, but if it were practiced, it would fall within sociocultural norms or acceptable practices.
- **Do they have a low frequency rate?** Do the behaviors require a rate of performance that makes them fit easily into a person's daily routine?
- **Are they of short duration or require little persistence?**

- **Do they have low cost?** Costs may include time, energy, or social-status costs, as well as financial or material costs.
- **Do they have approximations?** Are desired behaviors similar to those the person is already performing?
- **Are they not too complex,** and can they be easily divided into a small number of elements or steps?
- **Are they readily observable** by an outside evaluator?

For each category, a behavior is assigned a value from 0 to 5, depending on whether the behavior demonstrates none of the criteria (score of 0) up to all the criteria (score of 5). For example, for positive consequences, 0 means that performing the behavioral step produces no positive consequences that can be perceived by the person performing it, and 5 means that performing the behavior produces major, easily perceived consequences. Scores from the nine categories are added, and the behaviors with the highest total scores are those to be considered as reasonable target behaviors.

Health Impact of the Behavior

0 No impact on health problem
2 Some impact
3 Significant impact
4 Very significant impact
5 Eliminates the health problem

Complexity of the Behavior

0 Unrealistically complex
1 Involves a great many elements
2 Involves many elements
3 Involves several elements
4 Involves few elements
5 Involves one element

Positive Consequences of the Behavior

0 None that mother could perceive
1 Few perceptible consequences
2 Some consequences
3 Significant consequences
4 Very significant consequences
5 Major perceptible consequences

Frequency of Behavior

0 Must be done at unrealistically high rate to achieve any benefit
1 Must be done hourly
2 Must be done several times each day
3 Must be done daily
4 May be done every few days
5 May be done occasionally and still have significant value

Cost of Engaging in the Behaviors

0 Requires unavailable resources or demands unrealistic effort
1 Requires very significant resources or effort expenditure
2 Requires significant resources or effort
3 Requires some resources or effort
4 Requires few resources or little effort
5 Requires only existing resources

Persistence

0 Requires compliance over an unrealistically long period of time
1 Requires compliance over a very substantial period of time
2 Requires compliance for a week or more
3 Requires compliance for several days
4 Requires compliance for a day
5 Can be accomplished in a brief time

Compatibility with Existing Practices

0 Totally incompatible
1 Very significant incompatibility
2 Significant incompatibility
3 Some incompatibility
4 Little incompatibility
5 Already widely practiced

Observability

0 Cannot be observed by an outsider
1 Is very difficult to observe
2 Is difficult to observe
3 Is observable
4 Is readily observable
5 Cannot be missed

Approximations Available

0 Nothing like this is done now
1 An existing practice is slightly similar
2 An existing practice is somewhat similar
3 An existing practice is similar
4 Several existing practices are similar
5 Several existing practices are very similar

Source: Adapted with permission from Green, Kreuter, Deeds, & Partridge, 1980, p. 61.

F. SELECTING TARGET BEHAVIORS: TARGET BEHAVIOR SELECTION WORKSHEETS

This methodology (adapted from Mata, 1992) was successfully used in a Peruvian communication program. It involves completing three sets of worksheets:

The **Technically Ideal Behavioral Profile** worksheet is the description of the medically prescribed behavioral steps necessary to carry out the health practice correctly.

The **Existing Behavioral Profile** worksheet is the description of the target's audience behaviors, identified through research during assessment.

The **Target Behavioral Profile** is the list of minimum behavioral steps that are feasible for the target audience to perform and are necessary to have impact on the health problem.

Each worksheet is organized into five columns: the behavior, the reason for performing it, its "cost," the benefit (or consequence) for performing it, and the vocabulary used to describe the behavior. As with the Behavior Analysis Scale, this process is not a scientifically rigorous methodology, but it assists the planning team in organizing its discussion.

To select the target behaviors using this methodology, the interdisciplinary planning team does the following:

1. Reviews the list of potential ideal behaviors and fills out the Ideal Behavioral Profile worksheet.
2. Reviews the secondary and primary research collected during assessment and fills out the Existing Behavioral Profile worksheet.
3. Selects target behaviors:
    a. Reviews the Ideal Behavioral Profile worksheet and eliminates all the behaviors and behavioral steps that do not have any demonstrated impact on the *health problem being addressed by the program.*

b. Compares the Ideal and Existing Behavioral Profile worksheets and identifies where the behaviors are the same. Transfers these behaviors to the Target Behavioral Profile worksheet.

c. Compares the Ideal and Existing Behavioral Profile worksheets and identifies where the target audience is performing approximations to the ideal behavior. Transfers the ideal behavior to the Target Behavioral Profile worksheet. The communication strategy will focus on how to shape the existing approximation to the ideal.

d. Identifies where actual behaviors are radically different from the ideal behaviors and analyzes why. There are two fundamental reasons why the target audience is not performing the target behaviors: it does not have the skills necessary to perform them (skills deficit), or environmental factors do not support and maintain them (performance deficit). If the absence of desired behaviors is due to a skills deficit, include them in the Target Behavioral Profile worksheet. The communication program will focus on teaching those new skills to the target audience. However, if the absence of target behaviors is due to a performance deficit, the interdisciplinary team should analyze the following:

- **Do the ideal behaviors have negative consequences** to the person performing them?
- **Are the ideal behaviors incompatible** with what the person is already doing or with sociocultural norms or acceptable practices?
- **Do the ideal behaviors require an unrealistic rate of frequency?**
- **Do the ideal behaviors require an unrealistic duration?**
- **Do the ideal behaviors have too high a cost in time, energy, social status, money, or materials needed to perform them?**
- **Are the ideal behaviors too complex and not easily divided into a small number of elements or steps?**

If the absence of desired behaviors is due to any of these criteria, do not include them in the Target Behavioral Profile. However, in some instances some of the remaining ideal behaviors are necessary to have a health impact. In this case, the team should analyze if there is an intermediate point between the ideal and the existing behavior which could still have some health impact. That point should be negotiated with the medical specialist. The "negotiated" behavior should be included in the Target Behavioral Profile worksheet.

4. Organizes the target behaviors into the sequence necessary to perform them correctly.
5. Assigns the behaviors to the various phases of the communication program in order of priority.

TECHNICALLY IDEAL BEHAVIORAL PROFILE

Ideal Behaviors	Reasons	Benefits They Offer	Price	Vocabulary

EXISTING BEHAVIORAL PROFILE

Existing Behaviors	Reasons for doing them	Benefits They Offer	Price	Problems	Vocabulary

TARGET BEHAVIORAL PROFILE

Target Behavior	Price	Benefits	Vocabulary

G. PLANNING FOR BEHAVIOR CHANGE CHECKLIST

I. SELECTING TARGET BEHAVIORS

____ List of target behaviors is a limited number that is manageable to introduce considering the time frame and resources of the communication program.

____ All behaviors that are **not necessary** to have an impact on this specific health problem have been eliminated.

____ All the target behaviors that are **not feasible** for the target audience to perform have been eliminated.

____ Communicators have taken existing approximations of the ideal behaviors into account in the selection of target behaviors.

____ Behaviors have been assigned to different phases of the communication program according to their priority.

____ An interdisciplinary team selected the target behaviors.

____ If a medical specialist was not a member of the interdisciplinary team, he or she has been consulted concerning the selection of target behaviors that have a demonstrated impact on the health problem.

II. SELECTING COMMUNICATION STRATEGIES

____ Communicators determined whether the absence or incorrect performance of the behaviors is a skills or performance deficit.

SKILLS DEFICIT

____ If the absence or incorrect performance of the target behaviors is due to a skills deficit, communicators have designed a strategy that will provide training and teach the skills necessary to perform the target behaviors correctly.

____ If the target audience is performing approximations to the target behavior, the communicators have designed a strategy that will reward these approximations while teaching correct frequency, duration, accuracy, and timing.

PERFORMANCE DEFICIT

____ If performance of the target behaviors is immediately punishing, the communicators have designed a strategy to decrease unpleasant consequences and/or increase more positive ones.

____ If performance of the target behaviors has no immediate results, the communicators have designed a strategy to introduce new positive consequences for behavior.

____ If other behaviors are more rewarding than the target behaviors, communicators have designed a communication strategy to increase rewards for the target behavior.

____ The consequences introduced or strengthened through communication strategies are those that are the most relevant, salient, culturally appropriate, and immediate to the **target audience,** as identified through research with these populations.

____ If the communication strategy introduces planned consequences, communicators have also designed antecedent strategies to increase the saliency of these consequences.

____ If the communication strategy introduces planned consequences, the communicators have determined how these consequences will be phased out over time and what more naturally occurring consequences will take their places.

III. SELECTING COMMUNICATION CHANNELS

____ Communicators have selected multiple communication channels, building on the strength of each one.

____ Communicators have used channels to provide and/or strengthen consequences, as well as antecedents.

Communicators have used channels to:

____ Provide pleasant consequences for the target behavior

____ Lower negative consequences to engaging in the target behaviors

____ Increase the saliency of consequences

H. TRAINING FOR BEHAVIOR CHANGE CHECKLIST

ANTECEDENTS
PREPARATION

____ Participants' needs are assessed.
____ Participants' skills are observed for planning purposes.
____ Observable objectives are established for each skill area.
____ Complex skills are broken down into discrete, manageable, and measurable steps.
____ The training schedule provides enough time so that participants can practice skills until they are fluent.
____ Terminology and procedures are standardized throughout the training session.

INSTRUCTIONS

____ Trainer explains in detail the desired behavior(s)/skills(s).
____ Trainer provides reasons or has trainees define reasons why they should care about what they are to learn.

DEMONSTRATION

____ Trainer demonstrates the behavior/skills and provides a model that can be observed and imitated.
____ Trainer asks trainees to say what is right about the demonstration.
____ Trainer demonstrates a model of inappropriate behavior/skill and asks trainees to say what is wrong.

BEHAVIOR
PRACTICE

____ The learning situation for practice is realistic, as similar as possible to the real-life situation in which the trainee will be performing the skills.

____ Trainees practice performing the behavior/skill until they are fluent.

CONSEQUENCES

FEEDBACK AND REINFORCEMENT

____ Trainees receive response-specific reinforcing feedback on what they did correctly during the practice session.

____ Trainees receive response-specific (rather than personal) reinforcing feedback on approximations to the target behaviors/skills.

____ Trainees received response-specific (rather than personal) correcting feedback on what they need to do differently in their next practice session.

BEHAVIORAL ASSIGNMENTS

____ Trainees are given a specific, measurable assignment to perform before the next training session/meeting/visit, based on the behavioral objectives of training.

____ Trainees describe and/or demonstrate their assignment at the beginning of the next training session/meeting/visit.

____ Trainees receive response-specific reinforcing feedback on what they did correctly during their homework.

____ Trainees receive response-specific (rather than personal) reinforcing feedback on approximations to the target behaviors/skills they performed during their homework.

____ Trainees received response-specific (rather than personal) correcting feedback on what they need to do to improve their homework the next time.

I. MONITORING FOR BEHAVIOR CHANGE CHECKLIST

GENERIC CHECKLIST

____ 1. Define monitoring in terms of specific target behaviors and behavioral steps necessary to have an impact on the health problem.

____ 2. Conduct observation of people performing the target behaviors and/or

____ 3. Review clinic records to observe less skill-dependent behaviors, such as timely immunizations and ORS packet distribution.

____ 4. Graph the monitoring data.

____ 5. Communicate monitoring data to people performing the behaviors, using the data as feedback to reward and maintain desired behaviors.

____ 6. Fine-tune the communication/training strategy based on the results of the monitoring data.

HEALTH WORKER'S INTERPERSONAL COMMUNICATION SUPERVISION CHECKLIST

____ 1. Define health worker's interpersonal communication in terms of specific target behaviors and behavioral steps that should be performed for effective interpersonal communication.

____ 2. Observe the health worker's interpersonal communication with several mothers and apply a performance checklist of the target behaviors.

____ 3. Graph the data from the observations.

____ 4. Discuss the data with the health worker.

____ 5. Praise the health worker for the specific behavior steps performed correctly.

____ 6. Correct specific behaviors the health worker needs to work on to improve interpersonal communication.

____ 7. Ask the health worker to practice these skills in simulations.

____ 8. Repeat steps 5 and 6 until the health worker is practicing these skills fluently.

____ 9. Ask the health worker for problems he or she might have in carrying out all of the steps necessary for effective interpersonal communication.

____ 10. Brainstorm with the health worker for solutions to these problems.

____ 11. Support the health worker in the specific actions necessary to implement these decisions.

References

Abrams, D. & Elder, J. (1986). Social learning principles for organizational health promotion: An integrated approach. In M. Cataldo & T. Coates (Eds.), *Health and industry: A behavioral medicine perspective* (pp. 28-51). New York: Wiley.

Academy for Educational Development. (1987). *Communication planning for child survival programs.* Washington, DC: Academy for Educational Development.

Baer, D., Wolf, M., & Risley, T. (1968). Some current dimensions of applied behavior analysis. *Journal of Applied Behavior Analysis, 1,* 91-97.

Bandura, A. (1977). *Social learning theory.* Englewood Cliffs, NJ: Prentice-Hall.

Barlow, D., Hayes, S., & Nelson, R. (1984). *The Scientist practitioner.* Elmsford, NY: Pergamon Press.

Baume, C. (1988). *HealthCom preliminary report on the results from the 1987 resurvey in Honduras.* Menlo Park, CA: Applied Communication Technology.

Baume, C. (1990). *The HealthCom resurvey of oral rehydration therapy practices in Honduras.* Menlo Park, CA: Applied Communication Technology.

Becker, M. H. (Ed.). (1974). The Health Belief Model and personal health behavior. *Health Education Monographs, 2,* 324–473.

Becker, M. H. (1979). Psychosocial aspects of health-related behavior. In H. E. Freeman & S. Levine (Eds.), *Handbook of medical sociology* (3rd ed.). Englewood Cliffs, NJ: Prentice-Hall.

Bentley, M. (1988). The household management of childhood diarrhea in rural North India. *Social Science and Medicine, 27*(1), 75–78.

Booth, E. (1985). AMA-MAS: A radio course on breastfeeding. In *Field Notes* (pp. 46–59). Washington, DC: HealthCom, Academy for Educational Development.

Debus, M. (1988). *Handbook for excellence in focus group research.* Washington, DC: Academy for Educational Development.

Eiseman, T. O., Patel, V. L., & Sena, S. O. (1987). Uses of formal and informal knowledge in the comprehension of instructions for oral rehydration therapy in Kenya. *Social Science Medicine, 25,* 1225–1234.

Elder, J. P., Boddy, P., Barriga, P., Aguilar, A. L., & Espinal, H. (1991). La experiencia hondureña en el control de las infecciones respiratorias agudas infantiles. *Boletín de la Oficina Sanitaria Panamericana,* 110(5), 390–401.

Elder, J., Geller, E., Hovell, M., & Mayer, J. (in press). *Motivating health behavior.* Albany, NY: Delmar.

Elder, J. P., Louis, T., Sutisnaputra, O., Sulaeiman, N. S., Ware, L., Shaw, W., de Moor, C., & Graeff, J. A. (1992). The use of diarrhoeal management counselling cards for community health volunteer training in Indonesia: The HealthCom Project. *Journal of Tropical Medicine and Hygiene, 95*(5), 301–308.

Elder, J., Pratdesaba, M. E., Pineda, O. P., (1988–89). A behavior analysis of the promotion of oral rehydration therapy (ORT) in Guatemala. *International Quarterly of Community Health Education, 9*(2), 139–150.

Fishbein, M., & Ajzen, I. (1975). *Beliefs, attitudes, intention, and behavior: An introduction to theory and research.* Reading, MA: Addison-Wesley.

Fishbein, M., & Ajzen, I. (1980). *Understanding attitudes and predicting social behavior.* Englewood Cliffs, NJ: Prentice-Hall.

Freeman, H. E., & Levine, S. (Eds.). (1989). *Handbook of medical sociology*. (4th ed.). Englewood Cliffs, NJ: Prentice-Hall.

Galway, K., Wolff, B., & Sturgis, R. (1987). *Child survival: Risks and the road to health*. Columbia, MD: Institute for Resource Development/Westinghouse.

Geller, E. S., Johnson, R. P., & Pelton, S. L. (1982). Community-based interventions for encouraging safety belt use. *American Journal of Community Psychology, 10*, 138–195.

Geller, E., Lehman, G., & Kalsher, N. (1989). *Behavior analysis training for occupational Safety*. Newport, VA: Make-a-Difference, Inc.

Glanz, K., Lewis, F. M., & Rimer, B. K. (Eds.). (1990). *Health behavior and health education: Theory, research, and practice*. San Francisco: Jossey-Bass.

Goodman, R., & Steckler, A. (1990). Mobilizing organizations for health enhancement: Theories of organizational change. In K. Glanz, F. Lewis, & B. Rimer (Eds.), *Health behavior and health education: Theory, research and practice* (pp. 314–341). San Francisco: Jossey-Bass.

Green, L., & Kreuter, M. (1991). *Health promotion planning: An educational and environmental approach* (2nd ed.). Mountain View, CA: Mayfield.

Green, L., Kreuter, M. W., Deeds, S. G., Partridge, K. B. (1980). *Health education planning: A diagnostic approach*. Mountain View, CA: Mayfield.

Green, L., & Lewis, F. (1986). *Measurement and evaluation in health education and health promotion*. Mountain View, CA: Mayfield.

Gross, A., & Drabman, R. (1982). Teaching self-recording, self-evaluation and self-reward to nonclinic children and adolescents. In P. Karoly and F. Kanfer (Eds.), *Self management and behavior change*. Elmsford, NY: Pergamon Press.

Hersen, M., & Bellack, A. (Eds.). (1981). *Behavioral assessment*. Elmsford, NY: Pergamon Press.

Holland, J., & Skinner, B. (1961). *The analysis of behavior*. New York: McGraw-Hill.

Holmes, K., & Aral, S. O. (1991). Behavioral interventions in developing countries: In J. N. Aral & K. K. Holmes (Eds.), *Research issues in human behavior and sexually transmitted diseases in the AIDS era* (pp. 318–344). Washington, DC: American Association for Microbiology.

Hornik, R., Contreras-Budge, E., Ferencic, N., Koepke, C., & Morris, N. (1991). *Results from the evaluation of the PREMI/HealthCom project in Ecuador: 1985–1988*. Philadelphia: Center for International Health and Development Communication, Annenberg School for Communication, University of Pennsylvania.

Hornik, R., Zimicki, S., & Lee, M. (1991). *The HealthCom project in the Philippines: Final case study evaluation report*. Philadelphia: Center for International Health and Development Communication, Annenberg School for Communication, University of Pennsylvania.

Israel, R., Foote, D., & Tognetti, J. (1987). *Operational guidelines for social marketing projects in public health and nutrition*. Paris: Nutrition Education Programme, UNESCO.

Kanfer, F. H., and Saslow, G. (1969). Behavioral diagnosis. In C. M. Franks (Ed.). *Behavior therapy: Appraisal and status*. New York: McGraw-Hill.

Karoly, P., and Harris, A. (1986). Operant methods. in F. Kanfer & A. Goldstein (Eds.). *Helping people change* (2nd ed.). Elmsford, NY: Pergamon Press.

Kazdin, A. (1981). Behavioral observation. In M. Hersen & A. Bellack (Eds.), *Behavioral assessment,* (pp. 101–124). Elmsford, NY: Pergamon Press.

Kendall, C., Foote, D., & Martorell, R. (1983). Anthropology, communications and health: The Mass Media and Health Practices program in Honduras. *Human Organization, 42*(4), 353–360.

Krasner, L. (Ed.). (1980). *Environmental design and human behavior: A psychology of the individual in society*. Elmsford, NY: Pergamon Press.

Kyenkya-Isabirye, M., & Magalheas, R. (1990). The mothers' support group role in the health care system. *International Journal of Gynecology and Obstetrics, 31*(suppl. 1), 85–90.

LeFebvre, R. (1990). Strategies to maintain and institutionalize successful programs: A marketing framework. In N. Bracht (Ed.), *Health promotion at the community level* (pp. 94–132). Newbury Park, CA.: Sage.

McDivitt, J., & McDowell, J. (1991). *Results from the Evaluation of the HealthCom project in Central Java, 1988–1989*. Philadelphia: Center for International Health and Development Communication, Annenberg School for Communication, University of Pennsylvania.

McGuire, W. J. (1964). Inducing resistance to persuasion: Some contemporary approaches. In L. Berkowitz (Ed.), *Advances in experimental social psychology* (Vol. 1). (pp. 79-98). San Diego, CA: Academic Press.

McKinley, J. (1976). Social network influences on morbid episodes and the career of help seeking. In L. Eisenbert & A. Kleinmanj (Eds.), *The relevance of social science for medicine*. Boston: Reidel.

Mager, R., and Pipe, P. (1984). *Analyzing performance problems* (2nd ed.). Belmont, CA.: Lake.

Mata, J. I. (1992). *CTTA: A method for the transfer of agricultural technology*. Washington, DC: Academy for International Development.

Miller, L. (1980). *Principles of everyday behavior analysis*. Pacific Grove, CA: Brooks/Cole.

Nelson, R., & Hayes, S. (1981). Nature of behavioral assessment. In M. Hersen & A. Bellack (Eds.), *Behavioral assessment*. (pp. 3–37). Elmsford, NY: Pergamon Press.

Novelli, W. (1990). Applying social marketing to health promotion and disease prevention. In K. Glanz, F. Lewis, B. Rimer (Eds.), *Health behavior and health education: Theory, Research, and Practice* (pp. 285-314). San Francisco: Jossey-Bass.

Pelto, G. (1991). The role of behavioral research in the prevention and management of invasive diarrheas. *Reviews of Infectious Diseases, 13* (suppl. 4), S255–S258.

Pillsbury, B. (1990). *Immunization: The behavioral issues*. Washington, DC: Office of Health/International Health and Development Associates, United States Agency for International Development.

Porter, D., Verzosa, C., Graeff, J., & Bagasao, T. (1992). *The ability of Philippine mothers to observe ARI signs in their children: An observational study*. Washington, DC: HealthCom, Academy for Educational Development.

Prochaska, J. (1979). *Systems of psychotherapy: A transtheoretical analysis.* Belmont, CA: Dorsey Press.

Rasmuson, M. (1985). Report on the 1982 "Happy Baby Lottery." In *Field Notes* (Project Brochure). Washington, DC: HealthCom, Academy for Educational Development.

Rasmuson, M., & Booth, E. (1985). The role of formative evaluation in the Mass Media and Health Practices Project." In *Field Notes* (pp. 84-91). Washington, DC: HealthCom, Academy for Educational Development.

Rasmuson, M., Seidel, R., Smith, W., & Booth, E. (1988). *Communication for child survival.* Washington, DC: Academy for Educational Development.

Reis, T., Elder, J., Satoto, Kodyat, B. A., & Palmer, A. (1990). An examination of the performance and motivation of Indonesian village health workers. *International Quarterly of Community Health Education, 11,* 19-27.

Rimm, D., & Masters, J. (1979). *Behavior therapy* (2nd ed.). San Diego, CA: Academic Press.

Rogers, E. (1973). *Communication strategies for family planning.* New York: Free Press.

Rogers, E., & Shoemaker, F. (1971). *Communication of innovations* (2nd ed.). New York: Free Press.

Rosenstock, I. M. (1974). Historical origins of the Health Belief Model. *Health Education Monographs, 2,* 328-335.

Rosenstock, I. M. (1977). What research in motivation suggests for public health. *American Journal of Public Health, 50,* 295-302.

Rotter, J. (1954). *Social learning and clinical psychology.* Englewood Cliffs, NJ: Prentice-Hall.

Sandler, J. (1986). Aversion methods. In F. Kanfer & A. Goldstein (Eds.), *Helping people change* (2nd ed.). (pp. 191-235). Elmsford, NY: Pergamon Press.

Seidel, R. (1992). *Results and realities: A decade of experience in communication for child survival.* Washington, DC: HealthCom, Academy for Educational Development.

Sircar, B. K., Deb, B. C., Sengupta, P. G., Mondal, S., Gupta, D. N., Sarkar, S., Sikder, S. N., Ghosh, S., Saha, N. C., & Pal, S. C. (1991). An operational study on implementation of oral rehydration therapy in a rural community of West Bengal, India. *Indian Journal of Medical Research, 93,* 297–302.

Smith, W. A. (1989). *Lifestyles for survival: The role of social marketing in mass education.* Washington, DC: Academy for Educational Development.

Smith, W. A., & Furst, B. G. (1986). The role of communication in reducing infant mortality due to diarrhea-related dehydration. *International Pediatrics, 1*(2), 120–122.

Sulzer-Azaroff, B., & Mayer, G. (1977). *Applying behavior analysis procedures with children and youth.* Troy, MO: Holt, Rinehart & Winston.

Touchette, P., Elder, J., & Nagiel, M. (1990). How much ORS solution is actually administered during home based therapy? *Journal of Tropical Medicine and Hygiene, 93,* 28–34.

United Nations. (1991). *World population prospects.* New York: United Nations.

United Nations Children's Fund (UNICEF). (1992). *The state of the world's children, 1992.* London: Oxford University Press.

United States Agency for International Development. (1991). *Child Survival, 1985–1990: A sixth report to Congress on the USAID program.* Washington, DC: United States Agency for International Development.

United States Department of Health and Human Services. (1989). *Making health communication programs work: A planner's guide.* Washington, DC: US Government Printing Office.

Verzosa, C., Bernaje, M., de Guzman, E., Hernandez, E., Reodica, C., & Taguiwalo, M. (1989). *Managing a communication program on immunization.* Washington, DC: Academy for Educational Development.

Werner, D., & Bower, B. (1982). *Helping health workers learn.* Palo Alto, CA.: Hesperian Foundation.

Windsor, R., Baranowski, T., Clark, N. & Cutter, G. (1984). *Evaluation of health promotion and education programs.* Mountain View, CA: Mayfield.

World Health Organization. (1986). *Guidelines for training community health workers in nutrition* (2nd ed.). Geneva: World Health Organization.

World Health Organization (1991). *EPI global overview.* Geneva:

World Health Organization, Expanded Programme on Immunization.

World Health Organization, Programme for Control of Acute Respiratory Infections. (1990). *Interim programme report.* Geneva: World Health Organization.

World Health Organization, Programme for control of Diarrheal Diseases. (1990). *Interim programme report.* Geneva: World Health Organization.

World Health Organization, Programme for Control of Diarrheal Diseases. (1991). *Guidelines for cholera control.* Geneva: World Health Organization.

World Health Organization, Programme for Control of Diarrheal Diseases. (in press). Geneva: World Health Organization.

Supplementary Reading

Bertrand, T. (1978). *Communication pretesting.* Chicago: Communication Laboratory, Community and Family Study Center, University of Chicago.

Booth, Elizabeth M. (1992). *Introduction to the design and production of educational and promotional radio materials.* Washington, DC: Academy for Educational Development.

Debus, M. (1988). *Handbook for excellence in focus group research.* Washington, DC: Academy for Educational Development.

Elkamel, F. (1986). *Developing communication strategies and programs.* Washington, D.C.: UNICEF.

Fine, S. H., (1990). *Social marketing: promoting the causes of public and nonprofit agencies.* Needham Heights, MA: Allyn & Bacon.

Frederiksen et al., (Eds.). (1984). *Marketing health behavior, principles, techniques, and applications.* New York: Plenum.

Green, L., & Kreuter, M. (1991). *Health promotion planning: An educational and environmental approach.* Mountain View, CA: Mayfield.

Griffithe, M. (1988). *Improving young child feeding during diarrhea: A guide for investigators and program managers.* Manoff

International, Inc., for PRITECH, Management Sciences for Health.

Mager, R. F. (1988). *Preparing instructional objectives* (2nd ed.). Belmont, CA: Lake Publishing Company.

Scrimshaw, S., & Hurtado, E. (1988). *Rapid assessment procedures (RAP) for nutrition and primary health programs.* Los Angeles: United Nations University and University of California.

Seidel, R. (1992). *Results and realities: A decade of experience in communication for child survival.* Washington, DC: Academy for Educational Development.

Surmanek, J. (1979). *Media planning: A practical guide.* National Textbook Company.

U.S. Department of Health and Human Services, National Institutes of Health. (1989). *Making health communication programs work: A planners guide.* (NIH Publication No. 89-1493). Bethesda, MD: Author.

U.S. Department of Health and Human Services, Public Health Service, National Institutes of Health, National Cancer Institute. (1984). *Making PSAs (public service announcements) work: A handbook for health communication professionals.* Bethesda, MD: Author.

U.S. Department of Health and Human Servives. (1984). *Pretesting in health communications: Methods, examples, and resources for improving health messages and materials.* Author.

Windsor, R. A., Baranowski, T., Clark, N., and Cutter, G. (1984). *Evaluation of health promotion and education programs.* Palo Alto, CA: Mayfield.

World Health Organization. (1987). *Communication: A guide for managers of national diarrhoeal disease control programmes.* Geneva: Author.

Zimmerman, et al. (1989). *Developing health and family planning print materials for low-literate audiences: A guide.* Program for Appropriate Technology in Health.

Index

A

A-B-C (antecedent-behavior-consequence) chain: antecedent/consequence two-stage sequence, 31–32; and communication channels, 85–89; defined, 31; and health communication, 31–33; linkages, 32–33; and power of consequences, 32; and training, 105; *See also* Antecedents; Behavior; Consequences
Abrams, D., 138
Academy for Educational Development (AED), 2, 11, 144
Acute respiratory infections (ARI): child mortality rate, 7; Honduran program, 47–48; and target behavior selection, 68; treatment, 7
Aguilar, A. L., 17
AIDS, and child survival, 3
Ajzen, I., 21
Anemia, 8
Antecedents: and applied behavior analysis, 27; and consequences, 31–32; and monitoring, 139–141; naturally occurring vs. planned, 27; and training, 105. *See also* A-B-C (antecedent-behavior-consequence) chain
Applied behavior analysis: and antecedents, 27; and behavioral complexity, 152; and consequences, 27–30; defined, 14–15; and negative reinforcement, 28; and social learning theory, 26–27; and target behavior, 30–31; terms, 27–36; usefulness, 17, 150–151. *See also* Behavior analysis
Approximations: breast-feeding example, 33–34; defined, 33; and maintenance, 139–141; and skills deficits strategies, 74–75
Aral, S. O., 3
Assessment, behavioral: and A-B-C (antecedent-behavior-consequence) chain, 39–40; and behavior observation, 49–50; and formative research, 44–46; and health communication pro-

grams, 37–38; and health practice analysis/"ideal" behavior definition, 38–43; questions, 38; and secondary research review, 44; skills, questions, 96–97; steps, 38–46. *See also* Evaluation; Observation, behavior

B

Baer, D., 14, 28, 77, 90
Bandura, A., 24, 27, 71, 90, 101
Barlow, D., 52, 55, 58
Barriga, P., 17
Baume, C., 17, 146
Becker, M. H., 20
Behavior: and A-B-C chain, 31–32; and applied behavior analysis, 30–31; and approximations, 33–34; Communication/Persuasion Model, 21; competing, 31, 152; complexity, 31, 152; Diffusion of Innovations model, 23; Health Belief Model, 20; "ideal," 37, 38–43; models, 19–27; and planned antecedents, 27; Precede/Proceed Model, 23; and social learning theory, 24–27; and Theory of Reasoned Action, 21; Transtheoretical Model, 21–23. *See also* A-B-C (antecedent-behavior-consequence) chain; "Ideal" behavior; Target behavior
Behavior analysis: and approximations, 33–34; characteristics of programs applying, 35–36; and fading, 34; and health communication, 16; and health practices, 133–134; and learning vs. maintenance conditions, 35; misconceptions, 16–17, 150; principles, 15–16; and shaping, 34, 151; and skills/performance deficits, 34; stepwise approach, 151. *See also* Applied behavior analysis
Behavior Analysis Scale, 69, 80, 151
Behavior assessment. *See* Assessment, behavioral
Behavior change. *See* Change, behavior
Behavior change maintenance/monitoring. *See* Maintenance, health practice; Monitoring, behavior change
Behavior observation/selection. *See* Observation, behavior; Selection, behavior
Behavioral products observation: growth-monitoring example, 56–57; oral rehydration salts usage example, 55–56; practice, 55
Bellack, A., 39
Bernaje, M., 13, 138
Blindness, and vitamin A deficiency, 8
Boddy, P., 17
Booth, E., 14, 37, 48, 59, 79, 135
Bower, B., 71
Breast feeding/weaning: approximations example, 33–34; and child nutrition, 2, 8; and communication strategies, 76; and home/clinic trial observation, 56, 58; initiation/maintenance example, 135; performance deficit example, 72

C

"Catch them doing something right," 102, 151. *See also* Positive reinforcement
Central Java, Indonesia, health care volunteers example, 77–78
Change, behavior: and behavior observation, 49; and behavior selection, 64; and communication, 13, 19, 110; cross-cultural applicability of, 151; future applications/directions of, 153–155; health care professionals' experience of, 150–153; monitoring, 109–130; reinforcing/maintaining, 117–129
Checklists: HealthCom West Java project, 94–95; monitoring, 112–

113; performance observation, 50. *See also* Forms
Child health/survival. *See* Health, child; Survival, child
Cholera, 5-6
Clinical records, 114-115
Communication: and assessment, 37; and behavior analysis, 16; and behavior change, 13, 19, 110; behavioral approach to, 1-2, 150-155; and child survival, 10-13; and consequences, 28-30; definition/goal, 13, 19, 110; and health behavior models, 19-27; interdisciplinary approach to, 14; and literacy rates, 3; and maintenance, 141-144; monitoring, activities, 143-144; programs and applied behavior analysis for, 35-36; research/action, 13-14; strategy development for, 44, 70-81. *See also* Communication channels; Communication programming; Communication strategies; Communicators
Communication channels: broadcast, 81; combining, 81, 82-83; immunization example of, 85-89; interpersonal, 81; and maintenance, 142-143; print, 81-82; selection, 81-83
Communication/Persuasion Model, 21
Communication programming: and A-B-C chain, 32-33; and applied behavior analysis, 35-36; and communication channel selection/use, 81-83; and communication strategy selection, 70-81; and consequence design, 30; and infectious disease control, 2; and maintenance, 134-135; and target behavior selection, 60-70; and training, 90. *See also* Communication strategies; Planning
Communication strategies: and A-B-C chain, 85-89; and behavior selection, 70-81; breastfeeding example of, 76; as consequences, 83-85; decision-making approach to, 72-74; development of, 44; Guatemalan water/sanitation program example of, 79-81; health care volunteer example of, 77-78; and health practice maintenance, 141-143; and skills/performance deficits, 71-72, 74-79; for when behavior is approximated, 74-75; for when behavior is too complex/difficult/costly, 79; for when nonperformance is more rewarding, 78; for when other behaviors are more rewarding, 78-79; for when performance creates no immediate results, 77-78; for when performance is immediately punishing, 76; for when subjects are ignorant of how to perform behavior, 74
Communicators: and behavior selection, 63-64; and behaviorally focused communication program planning, 37-38, 46; and communication strategies, 70-79; and consequence application, 30; defined, 13; information collection techniques of, 44-45; and monitoring, 109-118; and positive reinforcement, 28, 143; role of, 13-14; and target behavior, 30-31
Consequences: abstract, 29; and antecedents, 31-32; and applied behavior analysis, 27-30; characteristics and health behavior and, 28-30; concrete vs. abstract, 29; and health communication programming, 30; importance of, 152-153; introducing new, 83-84; and maintenance programs, 46-47, 134, 139-141; naturally occurring, 29; negative, 84; planned, 29-30; positive, 110-111, 143, 153; power of, 32; and qualita-

tive/quantitative research, 46; saliency, 84-85; and training, 105. *See also* A-B-C (antecedent-behavior-consequence) chain
Contreras-Budge, E., 17
Convention on the Rights of the Child, 5

D

Debus, M., 44, 47, 50, 63
Deeds, S. G., 23, 69
de Guzman, E., 13, 138
Demonstration: and modeling, 99; Papua New Guinea oral rehydration therapy example of, 99-100; usefulness of, 99
Developing countries: cholera pandemic in, 5-6; health care overload in, 3; health care questions in, 3-4; health communication and child survival in, 11; health-related demographics in, 2-3; literacy rates in, 3
Diarrheal diseases: behavior observation example of, 95-96; and child mortality rate, 5; control and training sequence for, example of, 106-107; Honduran, control program for, 40-41, 144-148; self-monitoring of training example for, 126-127. *See also* Oral rehydration therapy (ORT)
Diffusion of Innovations model, 23
Direct observation, 114
Duration recording: immunization example of, 54-55; practice of, 54

E

Eiseman, T. O., 46
Elder, J. P., 14, 17, 19, 55, 56, 71, 78, 138, 139
Environment, and public health, 155
Espinal, H., 17
Ethnographic study, 45
Evaluation: and behavior change, 111-113; of health care workers, 94-95; literature about, 113; and monitoring, 111-112. *See also* Assessment, behavioral
Expanded Programme of Immunization (EPI), 6, 85

F

Fading, 34
Family planning, 3
Feedback/reinforcement: constructive, 102-103, 110-111; criteria, 102; critical dimensions of, 101-102; and feedback loops, 128-129; monitoring data use for, 117-129; and skill selection, 102. *See also* Negative reinforcement; Positive reinforcement
Ferencic, N., 17
Fishbein, M., 21
Focus group discussion, 45, 50
Foote, D., 38
Formative research, 44
Forms: behavioral observation, 59-60; Ideal Behavioral Profile worksheet, 70; Target Behavior Selection Worksheet, 70. *See also* Checklists; Graphs
Frequency recording: feeding/oral rehydration salt administration example of, 53-54; practice of, 53
Furst, B. G., 37

G

The Gambia oral rehydration therapy, 48-49
Geller, E. S., 14, 19, 103
Graphs: behavioral observation, 61; and feedback, 117-129; and feedback loops, 128-129; and monitoring, 115-117. *See also* Forms
Green, L., 23, 69
Growth monitoring, and behavioral products observation, 56-57
Guatemala: feeding during diar-

rhea study in, 69; water/sanitation case study in, 42–43, 68, 79–81

H

Harris, A., 28
Hayes, S., 30, 52, 55, 58
Health, child: and acute respiratory infections, 7; and AIDS, 3; and anemia, 8; and blindness, 8; and child nutrition, 7–9; demographics and, 2–3; and diarrheal disease control, 5–6; and family planning, 3; and high-risk fertility, 10; and immunizable diseases, 6–7; and infectious diseases, 2; international conference goals for, 4–10; and malaria, 9–10; and mental retardation, 8; and micronutrient deficiency, 2–3, 8–9
Health Belief Model, 20
Health care professionals/volunteers. *See* Professionals, health care; Volunteers, health care
Health care workers: evaluation of, 94–95; and mothers feedback loop, 128; and supervisor feedback loop, 128; as trainers, 91, 100. *See also* Volunteers, health care
Health communication/communicators. *See* Communication; Communicators
Health communication programming. *See* Communication programming
Health practice maintenance. *See* Maintenance, health practice
Health worker–mother feedback loop, 128
HealthCom: and behavior analysis principles, 16–17; and child health goals, 5; project description, 11–13; title change of, 11; West Java project checklist for, 94
Hernandez, E., 13, 138
Hersen, M., 39
High-risk fertility: and child mortality rate, 10; and family planning, 3
Holland, J., 27, 33, 49
Holmes, K., 3
Home/clinic trial observation: practice of, 56; weaning food preparation example of, 56, 58
Homework: and feedback, 103–104; mothers' skills training example of, 104–105
Honduran Diarrheal Disease Control Program: antecedent strategy (messages for), 145; and communication issues, 147; and health care delivery system, 145; "ideal" behavior for oral rehydration therapy example in, 40–41; and maintenance, 147–148; media mix for, 146; national project for, 144; pilot project for, 144; and programmatic issues, 147–148; supporting events for, 145–147; target behavior for, 144–147
Honduras: acute respiratory infection program in, 47–48; immunization and narrative recording example in, 51–53. *See also* Honduran Diarrheal Disease Control Program
Hornick, R., 17
Hovell, M., 14, 19

I

"Ideal" behavior: and behavior selection, 65; defining, 37, 39, 65; and Guatemalan water/sanitation case study, 42–43; oral rehydration therapy example for, 40–41; and vitamin A example, 65; worksheet, 70. *See also* Target behavior
Ideal Behavior Profile worksheet, 70
Immune system, and malnutrition, 7–8

Immunizable diseases: child mortality rate for, 6; and Expanded Programme of Immunization, 6; obstacles to prevention of, 6–7. *See also* Immunization; Infectious diseases
Immunization: and antecedents, 27; and communication channels, 85–89; duration recording example for, 54–55; and measles, in Philippines, 64; narrative recording example for, 51–53. *See also* Immunizable diseases
In-depth interview, 45, 50
Infectious diseases: and global issues, 155; and malnutrition, 2. *See also* Immunizable diseases
Information, education, and communication (IEC), 13
Instructions: defined, 97–98; presentation of, 98
Iodine: deficiency, 8; supplementation, 2–3, 8
Iron: deficiency, 8; supplementation, 3, 8
Israel, R., 38

K

Kalsher, N., 103
Kanfer, 37
KAP (knowledge, attitudes, and practices) studies, 44, 46
Karoly, P., 28
Kazdin, A., 49, 52
Kendall, C., 38
Knowledge, attitudes, and practices (KAP) studies, 44, 46
Koepke, C., 17
Krasner, L., 134
Kreuter, M. W., 23, 69
Kyenkya-Isabirye, M., 72

L

Learning: and maintenance conditions, 35; stepwise approach to, 134; vicarious, 24, 101. *See also* Social learning theory
Lee, M., 17
Lehman, G., 103
Lesotho, oral rehydration therapy study, 55
Literacy, and health communication, 3

M

McDivitt, J., 17
McDowell, J., 17
McGuire, W. J., 21
McKinley, J., 136
Magalheas, R., 72
Mager, R., 75
Maintenance, as health practice: and antecedents, 139–141; and approximations, 139–141; and behavioral principles, 133–134, 153; and communication channels, 142–143; and communication issues, 143–144; and communication program implications, 134–136; and communication strategies, 141–143; and consequences, 134, 139–141; and favorable environment, 134; Honduran oral rehydration therapy example for, 144–148; and initiation, 134–135; and skills/performance deficits, 141; support sources for, 136–139, 152
Malaria: child mortality rate from, 9; prevention/treatment of, 9–10
Malnutrition: child mortality rate from, 7; and immune system, 7–8; and infectious diseases, 2
Martorell, R., 38
Mass Media for Health Practices (MMHP), 11. *See also* HealthCom
Masters, J., 28, 33
Mata, J. I., 70
Mayer, G., 27, 33, 37, 39, 54, 71, 77, 134
Mayer, J., 14, 19
Media mix, 81, 82–83, 146
Mental retardation, and iodine deficiency, 8

Mexico, oral rehydration therapy study, 55
Micronutrient supplements, 2–3, 8
Miller, L., 27, 28, 32, 33, 53, 58, 61, 71, 77, 134
Ministry of Health (MOH): African, training program example of, 123–126; applying behavioral principles to, 153–154; and health workers-mothers feedback loop, 128–129; and HealthCom project, 12–13; and health communicator, 14; Latin American, communication program example of, 120–122
Momentary time sampling, 58
Monitoring, behavior change: as behavior, 129–130; and behavior selection, 113–114; and clinical records, 114–115; data collection for, 113–115; defined, 111–112; and direct observation, 114; and evaluation, 111–112; and feedback loops, 128–129; graphing data for, 115–117; health center utilization example of, 118–120; instruments for, 112–113; observers for, 61; oral rehydration therapy behavior change example of, 113–114; outside health clinic example of, 120–122; principles of, 110–111; in self, 115, 125–127; techniques for, 114–115; training outcomes of, 123–126
Morris, N., 17
Mortality: and acute respiratory infections, 7; and childhood diseases, 85; and diarrheal diseases, 5; and high-risk fertility, 10; and immunizable diseases, 6; and malaria, 9; and malnutrition, 7. *See also* Survival, child
Mothers: breast-feeding/weaning practices of, 2, 8, 56, 58, 72, 76, 135; and health workers feedback loop, 128; high-risk fertility behavior of, 3, 10; and malaria, 9; pregnant, and iodine deficiency, 8; training of, 91, 100, 104
Mumba Clinic, Africa, 118–120

N

Nagiel, M., 17, 55, 56
Narrative (A-B-C) recording: Honduran immunization example of, 52–53; practice of, 51–52
Naturally occurring antecedents, 27
Naturally occurring consequences, 29
Negative reinforcement, 28, 101. *See also* Consequences: negative; Feedback/reinforcement
Nelson, R., 30, 52, 55, 58
1990 World Summit for Children, 5
Novelli, W., 38
Nutrition: and breast feeding, 2, 8; and micronutrient supplements, 2, 8, 85
Nutrition Institute for Central America and Panama (INCAP), 42, 79

O

Observation, behavior: and behavior change, 49; and behavioral assessment, 49–50; and behavioral products observation, 55–56; diarrheal diseases workshop example of, 95–96; and duration recording, 54–55; forms for, 59–60; and frequency recording, 53–54; graphing results of, 61; and home/clinic trial observation, 56, 58; and narrative recording, 51–53; and observer selection/training/monitoring, 60–61; and performance observation, 50–51; and qualitative/quantitative research, 47–49; as research technique, 45–46; and self-report, 49; "snapshot," 58; structured, 50; systemic, 58–61; timing of, 58–59; and training program evaluation, 93–97; types of, 50–58. *See*

also Assessment, behavioral; Behavioral products observation; Home/clinic trial observation; Observers; Performance observation
Observers: monitoring, 61; selecting, 60; training, 60-61. *See also* Observation, behavior
Oral rehydration salts (ORS), 5, 31, 50-51, 53-54, 55-56, 100, 113-114, 143, 144
Oral rehydration therapy (ORT): and cholera, 6; and diarrheal diseases prevention, 5; and The Gambia, 48-49; and health care workers' evaluation, 95-96; Honduran, program in, 40-41, 144-148; and "ideal" behavior assessment, 40-42; Lesotho, study on, 55; Mexico, study on, 55; monitoring behavior change example of, 113-114; Papua New Guinea, program in, 99-100; procedure, 5; and qualitative/quantitative research techniques, 47, 48-49; skills practice example of, 100; and social learning theory, 26; training sequence example of, 106-107. *See also* Diarrheal diseases

P

Palmer, A., 78, 138
Papua New Guinea, oral rehydration therapy program in, 99-100
Partridge, K. B., 23, 69
Patel, V. L., 46
Pelto, G., 44
Performance observation: checklist for, 50; oral rehydration salts usage example of, 50-51
Philippines, measles immunization program in, 64
Pipe, P., 75
Planned antecedents, 27
Planned consequences, 29-30
Planning: of behaviorally focused communication program, 37-38, 46; of communication strategies, 141-143; and primary/secondary research results, 63. *See also* Communication programming
Positive reinforcement, 28, 101-102, 151. *See also* Consequences: positive; Feedback/reinforcement
Practice: defined, 100; oral rehydration therapy example of, 100
Precede/Proceed model, 23
Prochaska, J., 21
Professionals, health care: behavior change experience of, 150-153; and behavioral analysis, 17; in developing countries, questions of, 3-4; and future health care practices/directions, 153-155; and global issues, 154-155; and health care resources, 155
Psychology, operant, 26
Public health: and environmental issues, 155; and global issues, 154-155; international blueprint for, 4-5; resources and, 155; theory-based interventions in, 11; training opportunities in, 91-92

Q

Qualitative/quantitative research: and behavioral questions, 47-49; and consequences, 46; focus of, 46

R

Rasmuson, M., 14, 37, 48, 59, 135
Reinforcement. *See* Feedback/reinforcement; Negative reinforcement; Positive reinforcement
Reis, T., 78, 139
Reodica, C., 13, 138
Research: formative, 44; qualitative/quantitative, 46-49; secondary, 44; and target audiences, 44-45
Research assessment techniques: behavior observation, 45-46; eth-

nographic study, 45; focus group discussion, 45; in-depth interview, 45; survey, 45. *See also* Observation, behavior
Resources, public health, 155
Rimm, D., 28, 33
Risley, T., 14, 28, 77, 90
Rogers, E., 23
Rosenstock, I. M., 20
Rotter, J., 24

S

Sandler, J., 28
Sanitation, Guatemalan hand-washing case study, 42–43, 79–81
Saslow, 37
Satoto, Kodyat, B. A., 78, 138
Secondary research, 44
Seidel, R., 14, 37, 59, 64, 135
Selection, behavior: acute respiratory infection example of, 68; and assessment research, 65; and Behavior Analysis Scale, 69–70; and behavior change, 64; and elimination process, 67–68; and "ideal" behavior, 65; and monitoring, 113–114; short list for, 64, 69; steps for, 65–69; and Target Behavior Selection Worksheets, 70; and target behaviors, 65–69; tools for, 69–70
Self-efficacy, 24
Self-monitoring, 115, 126–127
Sena, S. O., 46
Shaping, 34
Shoemaker, F., 23
Skills/performance deficits: and approximate behavior, 75–76; breast-feeding example of, 72; and communication strategy selection, 71–72; defined, 34; differentiating between, 141; and ignorance, 74; strategies addressing, 74–79
Skills training: and deficits, 34; and demonstration, 99–100; and feedback/reinforcement, 101–103; for health care volunteers, 71; and homework, 103–105; and instructions, 97–98; and modeling, 99; monitoring communication example of, 123–126; Papua New Guinea oral rehydration example of, 99–100; and practice, 100–101; steps of, 97–105; worker skills checklist for, 94–95. *See also* Demonstration; Feedback/reinforcement; Homework; Instructions; Practice; Training
Skinner, B., 27, 33, 49
Smith, W. A., 14, 37, 59, 135
Social learning theory: and applied behavior analysis, 26–27; and operant psychology, 26; and oral rehydration skills, 26; and self-efficacy, 24; and vicarious learning, 24
Stages of Change Model, 21
Sulzer-Azaroff, B., 27, 33, 37, 39, 54, 71, 77, 134
Supervisor-health worker feedback loop, 128
Surveys, 45, 50
Survival, child: and acute respiratory infections, 7; and AIDS, 3; and diarrheal diseases, 5; and global health problems, 155; and health communication, 10–13; and high-risk fertility, 10; and human factor, 154; and immunizable diseases, 6; and malaria, 9; and malnutrition, 7. *See also* Mortality

T

Taguiwalo, M., 13, 138
Target audiences: and communication channels, 81; health practices assessment for, 38–42; and maintenance programs, 134–135; research techniques for surveying, 44–45
Target behavior: and approximations, 33; and consequences, 32, 83–84; considerations in evaluat-

ing, 30–31; defined, 65; and performance observation, 51; selection, 60–70; and skills/performance deficits, 34. *See also* Behavior; "Ideal" behavior
Theory of Reasoned Action, 21
Timing, 58–59
Tippy-Tap, 43, 80
Tognetti, J., 38
Touchette, P., 17, 55, 56
Training: and A-B-C (antecedent-behavior-consequence) chain, 105; as antecedent, 105; behavioral model of, 90–91; as consequence, 105; evaluation and behavior observation in, 93–97; of health care workers, 71, 91, 93; for behavior monitoring, 129; monitoring outcomes of, 123–126; of mothers, 91; of observers, 60–61; in public health programs, 91–92; as reinforcement, 105–107; sequence example of, 106–107; and skills assessment questions, 96–97. *See also* Skills training
Transtheoretical Model, 21–23

U

United Nations, 2, 5
United Nations Children's Fund (UNICEF), 4, 5, 44
United States Agency for International Development (USAID), 7, 8, 9, 10, 11, 44, 144
United States Department of Health and Human Services, 81, 82, 85

V

Verzosa, C., 13, 138
Vitamin A: and childhood diseases mortality, 85; deficiency of, 8–9; "ideal" behavior example related to, 65; supplementation of, 2, 8
Volunteers, health care: attrition of, 71, 77; and communication strategies, 77–78; training for, 71

W

Werner, D., 71
Wolf, M., 14, 28, 77, 90
Worksheets. *See* Forms
World Health Organization (WHO), 4, 6, 42, 44, 79
World Health Organization, Programme for Control of Diarrheal Diseases, 5, 6, 7, 126

Z

Zimicki, S., 17

The case study in Chapter Three, "Defining the Ideal Behavior in a Guatemalan Water and Sanitation Program," is used with the permission of Elena Hurtado (formerly of INCAP).

Photo Credits

The photo opening Chapter One is of a health worker conducting a prenatal visit in Burkina Faso, West Africa, and is from the collection of the Nutrition Communication Project, USAID Office of Nutrition, Washington, D.C.

The photo opening Chapter Two is of mothers learning treatment for diarrhea from flier and radio in The Gambia, West Africa, and is from the collection of the Mass Media and Health Practice Project.

The photo opening Chapter Three is of interdisciplinary team members washing hands during the assessment phase in Guatemala and was taken by Elizabeth Mills Booth. It is from the INCAP collection.

The photo opening Chapter Four is of a communicator pretesting a poster with a mother in Honduras and is from the HealthCom collection.

The photo opening Chapter Five is of a health clinic scene in the Philippines and was taken by José Raphael Hernandez, a staff member of the HealthCom Project there.

The photo opening Chapter Six is of a behavioral observation of a mother using the ORS mixing bag in Guatemala and was taken by John Elder.

The photo opening Chapter Seven is of a health worker instructing a mother on ORS mixing and administration in Honduras and is from the HealthCom collection.

The photo opening Chapter Eight is of three smiling children in Mali, West Africa, and is from the collection of the Nutrition Communication Project, USAID Office of Nutrition, Washington, D.C.